WHAT DOCTORS CANNOT TELL YOU

WHAT DOCTORS CANNOT TELL YOU

clarity, confidence and uncertainty in medicine

by Kevin B. Jones, M.D.

TALLOW
BOOK

Salt Lake City

For permission to reproduce selections from this book, please contact:
info@tallowbook.com

Publisher's Cataloging-in-Publication
(Provided by Quality Books, Inc.)

    Jones, Kevin B.
       What doctors cannot tell you : clarity, confidence
    and uncertainty in medicine / by Kevin B. Jones.
       p. cm.
       Includes bibliographical references.
       LCCN 2012934195
       ISBN 978-0-9852454-7-4
       ISBN 978-0-9852454-5-0 (eBook)
       ISBN 978-0-9852454-3-6

       1. Physician and patient.   I. Title.

   R727.3.J66 2012   610.69'6
                        QBI12-600060

Printed in the United States of America.

Illustrations by page number:
    p7 adapted from The Universal Compound Microscope, by B. Martin c.1760
    p34 Scene in the Practice of a New York Surgeon, by Edward H. Dixon, c.1855.
    p37 Explanatory sketch of bell curves by Kevin B. Jones.
    p49 Muscles and Bones of the Forearm and Hand, by Gerard de Lairesse, 1690.
    p68 La Consultation, by Charles Etienne Pierre Motte, c. 1830.
    p95 adpated from Amputation Instruments, by Jonas Arnold Delineavit, 1666.
    p96 Leaurelle Oil, advertisement from the Druggists' Circular, volume 34, 1890.
    p118 Golden Goose Ostrich, first presented in 1915 by Ernest Amory Codman.
    p150 A Pharmaceutical Lesson, by Hieronymus Brunschwig, 1500.
    p177 The Zodiac, a medieval woodcut from Europe, 16th century.
    p178 adapted from Oriatrike, Physick Refined, the title page from the 1662 book.
    p199 The Plague in 1665, by W. Sherlock in *History of England*.
    p220 *Surgite mortui venite ad Judicium* [Arise, dead one, and come to
        Judgment] by J.F. Desclassan, 1779, in *Dance of Death* by J. Gamelin.
    p242 adapted from Physician Struggling with Death for Life, by Ivo Saliger, 1920

        (voluntarily released to the public domain before 1973).

All illustrations are considered to be in the public domain. Originals for all but those
on p37, p118 and p177 are courtesy of the National Library of Medicine.

FOR my father,
who taught me that it is most important to be honest
when it is least convenient

and my patients,
who provide many opportunities to test this principle.

AUTHOR'S NOTE

The stories within this book are true, about real people.

To protect the anonymity of these patients and colleagues, I have changed many names as well as other identifying characteristics. Specifically, Drs. Smith, MacArthur, Roberts and Goldstein are fictitious names.

Further, this book hopes to advise all to engage the counsel of competent medical professionals, not replace their role in any reader's medical decision-making. The only medical advice this book offers is that you should ask questions of your physician.

Finally, the views represented in this book are my own and do not necessarily represent the opinion of the University of Utah, Huntsman Cancer Institute, or Primary Children's Medical Center, where I see patients and do research.

CONTENTS

PART 2: TREATMENT

PART 3: PROGNOSIS

PROLOGUE

I have only been fired by a patient once.

I think I know why.

I remember Carl, sitting there in the clinic room. He pressed his lips so firmly together that they blanched. His frustration was palpable. Although we faced each other, he no longer really looked at me. His eyes focused on a point beyond my shoulder.

I was losing him.

"Radiation begins next week," I said, reluctantly rising to leave the room. "I'll give you a call a week or so after that to see where you are on this surgical decision."

"That's fine," he answered, flatly.

But it wasn't fine. It was anything but fine.

I called him two weeks later.

Before I could say anything of substance, he asked quietly, "What do you think about a second opinion?"

"I think it's a great idea," I said. "I doubt anyone will have any different options to offer, but another surgeon will see your options differently. A new perspective may help your thinking. I'll set up an appointment for you with my partner."

Why didn't Carl want to see me again?

I was, he told my partner, "the guy who told him he might lose his leg."

Just so --- I *was* the guy who told him he might lose his leg.

What I also told him was that he might prefer amputation to the option that might save his leg.

I don't know if he heard that part.

Carl wasn't unhappy about anything I knew or didn't know. What I had or hadn't done didn't bother him. What I *told* him troubled him.

Should I not have told him?

Words wield incredible power. Even a single word can undo an entire conversation, especially if the word impacts one's health or that of a loved one.

Josh had a sore knee. He figured that it was his high school football injury flaring up two decades later. Still, he decided to have it checked, so he made an appointment with a sports medicine specialist. After describing his symptoms to the clinic nurse by telephone, she arranged an MRI to precede his visit with the surgeon.

After the MRI, Josh walked upstairs from the scanner to the waiting room of the sports clinic. He checked in, found a magazine from the rack. But before he could take a seat, the receptionist left her desk to speak to him.

"The doctor has already looked at the MRI," she began. "He wants to refer you to a Dr. Jones. Here's his contact information."

She handed Josh a post-it note on which she had neatly printed my name, my phone number and "Huntsman Cancer Institute."

Josh walked quietly out to his truck, the note clenched in his fist. He tried to call his dad, but got only voice mail. He sat there, stunned.

A few minutes passed. His cell phone rang.

"Hello?" he answered hesitantly.

"Hello," said a cheerful voice on the other end. "This is Michael at the Huntsman Cancer Institute. I understand that we need to set up an appointment for you to see Dr. Jones."

"Sure."

Not everyone who comes to see me as a patient at the Huntsman Cancer Institute has cancer. Although Josh didn't know it, the sports medicine specialist hadn't actually thought that cancer was his problem.

It didn't matter. The word had been spoken.

Spoken words, unspoken words --- they're equally powerful. When physicians leave blanks, patients fill them in. Some hear promises. Others hear threats.

It had been a full day of surgery for me. By the time I made my way over to the chemotherapy unit, it was nearly midnight. The late hour didn't matter. I had to try at least. Ewan's mother and I hadn't talked face-to-face since I called her the night before to relay her son's confirmed diagnosis of bone cancer.

While I had been in the OR with other patients, Ewan and his mother had met the chemotherapy team for admission to the hospital and begun the first dosing cycle. I doubted either would be awake after such a day. Ewan's mother had confessed by telephone the night before that she had slept little during the week since the biopsy. If neither were awake, I'd simply let the nurse know to tell them I had stopped by.

But Ewan's mother was awake. I found her sitting on the chair next to his bed, reading a folder of papers by flashlight. She quickly rose and ushered me back out to the hallway.

"He only fell asleep an hour ago," she explained in a whisper. "Let's talk out here."

"Out here will be fine. I don't need to check anything on Ewan anyway. I just came by to see how everything's going so far."

"Is this your cheerleader mode that you told me you would shift to now that Ewan is starting chemo?"

"That's right," I acknowledged. "Don't worry, though; I promise not to wear a skirt."

She smiled.

"I doubt I'd look very cute in one anyway. But yes, the chemo docs run this show for the next couple of months. I just cheer from the sidelines until the time comes for the big surgery."

"And that's at week 11, right?"

"Usually," I confirmed, shrugging my shoulders slightly.

"What do you mean by 'usually'?" she asked, concern unmasked in her voice. Without waiting for an answer, she plowed forward.

"This protocol says that Ewan will be here 3 days this week, then off two and half weeks, then here 5 days the next week, and 5 days the week after that, and then. . . . Oh wait, maybe I have that wrong," she interrupted herself, almost frantically flipping through her folder of papers.

I tried to reassure her.

"You have the protocol correct. Have you memorized it?"

"I just don't want to mess anything up. I don't want to miss anything." She seemed to be trying to brace herself. "Dr. Jones, you told Ewan and me that we win more often than we lose in cases like his, but not as often as you'd like. Today, I got the chemo protocol. It looks tough, but we can do it. I'll have to quit my job, but we can move in with my parents. I can do this. I will do anything for my Ewan. He's all I've got. I can follow this protocol to keep him safe."

I didn't tell her that her thinking was wrong --- I couldn't crush her belief that her obedience to this protocol would protect her precious boy. So my silence probably reinforced a promise she had heard in the unspoken words of the oncologist earlier in the day. Yes, I felt this regimen was the best available to manage Ewan's cancer. Yes, more children finishing this treatment course will survive than if not treated. Yes, she and Ewan should stick to the protocol as closely as possible. But obedience alone wouldn't save him.

I didn't choose to clarify that critical point.

I didn't tell her.

Few communications are more fraught than those between physicians and patients, no matter on which side of the white coat you find yourself.

But I am not your physician here.

So perhaps, here, I can tell you what your doctor can't tell you. And why he can't.

I will tell you about a physician who was literally run out of town for daring to suggest that medicine ought to keep track of results.

I will introduce you to a surgeon who dared not to operate.

I will explain how the muddle of disease and diagnosis and fuzzy biology sometimes creates a disconnect between doing right and getting it right.

I will tell you the story of a noble woman who took her chances and lost and another story of a frightened man who could not take a chance, but still lost.

You will meet a mother whose heart was breaking because her daughter had not yet died.

These are not, I want to emphasize, extraordinary cases.

These are not stories about beating the odds.

This is a book about ordinary cases and how extraordinarily difficult it is to be certain about the odds in the first place.

Here you will witness the rules of engagement and the space in which medical decisions are made.

What you won't see here: the brand of "differential diagnostics" as practiced by Hugh Laurie on the *House* TV series. That's because *House* is not, as they say, based on a true story. On the contrary, it's total fiction. A patient may hear a diagnosis from a single doctor, but rarely has that doctor arrived at the diagnosis alone. Diagnosis is a team sport. And like other team sports, it requires at least a modest ability to play well with others.

The lone genius with the repellent personality and a knack for plucking the right answer from the heavens --- that doctor doesn't exist. Here, we are dealing with people. On both sides of the space where decisions are made.

So the point of these stories isn't to encourage you to marvel at the skill of the people in the white coats. It's to help you learn to talk to your physician, how to understand what she or he says. And then it's to help you to ask your physician to invite you more fully into that privileged space, not as subject alone, but as *the* interested party.

Part One: Diagnosis

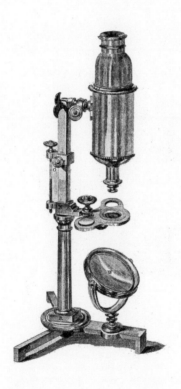

SATISFACTION OF SEARCH

Impenetrable

Sometimes a patient will answer my questions about his well-being with, "Aren't *you* supposed to tell *me* how I'm doing? *You're* the doctor."

Am I an auto mechanic?

If so, I am a poor one. I never got one of those magical little diagnostic computer devices that I could plug in to find out exactly what is wrong.

Or am I some sort of priest?

Well, that depends. The white coat ceremony certainly carried the gravity of a robing-in-the-cloth. Saying the Hippocratic oath sounded more like taking orders than graduating. But the real rite of induction occurred years earlier, when I walked through the doors into the gross anatomy lab during my first year of medical school. I was Moses, climbing Mount Horeb to witness the burning bush.[1]

I spent hours dissecting the peculiarly pickled human bodies. Pungent formaldehyde fumes permeated my skin, hair, and clothes. I obsessively washed my hands. I showered several times each day. Every effort failed to clear the air around me.

Descending from the Mount after repeat visits, Moses wore a veil to shield the Israelites from the brightness of his countenance.

My veil was a cloud of formaldehyde vapors. I maintained my distance whenever "down among the mere mortals" to keep from nauseating them.

From what did my veil protect them?

What secret had I witnessed within that inner sanctum behind the laboratory doors?

Was I really any brighter?

It is no secret that medical students dissect cadavers. People may be more aware of this course of study than of any other aspect of medical education. That is, aware that it happens. Aware of what it teaches? Definitely less so. Society limits such dissections to the hushed, reverent space behind those closed doors. Humanity has nearly always limited access to cadaveric dissections. The great artists of the Renaissance risked exile and torture for the opportunity to place their fingers on the dissection knife.

Cutting dead human flesh certainly takes some getting used to. There is an eerie, oozy, oily quality to it. But what does the exercise teach? The secrets from beneath the skin? Those cold, gray, formaldehyde-embalmed bodies answered none of *my* questions about what quivered beneath my own skin.

I recall thinking --- even as late as that first year of medical school --- that immediately beneath my skin was a lake of blood, ready to gush out at any provocation. I understood from physiology class that the total blood volume of the typical human body is only about five liters. And I understood that five liters could only fill the better part of one leg. Nonetheless, any cut I sustained on my finger or elsewhere immediately welled up with blood. This observation convinced me that my body must be comprised almost entirely of blood beneath the skin's surface.

Gross anatomy dissections of preserved bodies drained of blood could not solve the bleeding mystery. Despite having climbed the Mount and seen the bush, I saw no burning. Was it that life was missing? I awaited the next level: surgery. In my surgical rotation, surely I would see what really hid beneath the skin.

I remember watching my first large abdominal surgery as a medical student. It seemed almost irreverent; the surgeons quickly slashed open the enveloping tissues and pulled them apart with large hooks.

"Can it really be that simple?" I asked myself. "Can they just do that?"

Indeed it could, and they did.

There was no lake of blood inside.

After witnessing a few surgeries, I came to terms with it. Far from filled with blood, most tissue layers can be divided with very little bleeding. A dense network of tiny vessels weaves into the deeper layers of the skin, making it one of the bloodiest tissues in the body to divide. These vessels protect the mystery with a sudden gush of blood from a cut finger or a shaving mishap, but can be ignored in many surgical situations. This crimson flash wasn't the glimpse of a burning bush after all, only smoke and mirrors.

I can't count the number of times since then that my discussion of the risks, benefits, and uncertainties of a surgery has been dismissed by a patient or family member insisting that I will "just have to find out when I get in there." As a colloquial expression of the recognized uncertainty involved in any medical intervention, I appreciate the sentiment. What concerns me is that it also expresses some quiet belief that the diagnostic truths for the case lie under the skin, ready to be exposed by the first incision.

Very few surgeries are extensively guided by information gathered during the course of the surgery itself, after opening the skin. I gain more clarity on closing the skin than opening it. At the surgery's end I can easily check off answers to the pre-surgical unknowns: how long the surgery will take, how much the patient will bleed, or how well the patient will tolerate the anaesthetic. Very few uncertainties about diagnosis and its guidance of the overall treatment plan become clear when I open the skin.

The human skin is a barrier that few dare to violate. Having crossed it many times, I assure you that such crossings require neither priestly magic nor even great skill. There certainly remains nothing frightening or mysterious about it for me today. I rarely "find out when I get in there." When I get in there, I find exactly the same uncertainty lurking beneath the skin that I saw before cutting.

If physicians are priests, then we serve a yet hidden god. You might assume that anyone who has spent as many years in school as the typical physician *must* have learned something awfully fancy along the way. You will soon see, however, that learning --- and even knowing --- are, in medicine, not quite as clear as you might hope.

Near Miss

I met a teenager named Alana with her parents in the emergency room at our children's hospital. Alana had broken her femur during dance class. One of her classmates had accidentally kicked her mid-leap. Alana had fallen to the floor in pain.

X-rays in the ER plainly displayed destruction of a region of bone near the break in the mid thigh. I suspected a cancer had eaten the bone away, weakening it for the break. As it was late at night, Alana, her parents and I briefly reviewed our plan to get further information the next day. She needed an MRI of her femur and a biopsy.

Alana's mother followed me into the hall as I left to make these arrangements.

"You know, Dr. Jones, Alana's thigh has been hurting for nearly a year."

"Yes. She mentioned that."

"We kept trying to find out what it was," she continued. "She had x-rays and even an MRI. They thought it might be her hip, then maybe a pinched nerve in her spine. None of the tests showed anything. Could this have been there the whole time?"

"I don't know," I answered. "I expect that it was. Perhaps it was there, but not yet detectable."

"Alana isn't a complainer at all, but I eventually started trying to convince her to forget about it and get back to living. The doctor thought we had ruled out everything serious already. Even I had as good as given up on ever having an answer. Do you think they just missed something?"

"I doubt it, but even if they did, it's an easy thing to do. Even now the changes in Alana's bone are fairly subtle. A few months ago, they may have been imperceptible."

Alana's mother brought the prior imaging studies to me during the course of Alana's later cancer treatments. I found them instructive. All showed entirely normal anatomy. One was an MRI of Alana's spine. The other was a plain radiograph (what her mother called an "x-ray") of her hip. It was dated only five weeks prior to her fracture, not months.

In almost painful irony, the hip radiograph missed what was probably a visible portion of her tumor by no more than an inch. A femur radiograph rather than a hip radiograph --- or even a hip radiograph with a slightly larger field of view --- would have revealed the tumor a month earlier. Even more baffling, the tumor probably extended into the bone section visible on the hip radiographs, but didn't change the radiographic appearance of that part of the bone. A hip MRI, more discerning than the hip radiograph, would have shown this disease in the upper portion of the bone. The spine MRI that had been obtained, of course, didn't.

These other tests might have identified Alana's disease before the fracture did. Two expensive and technologically advanced imaging studies, only slightly misdirected, had failed to end the uncertainty of diagnosis in her case. If anything, they probably played a role in extending it. And having ordered expensive tests to no avail, Alana's physician and parents had grown reluctant to pursue more.

The spine MRI and hip radiographs were *ultimately* the wrong tests.

Both physicians and patients want to order the "correct" test, but each defines it in a different way.

The correct test from a physician's perspective will be based on protocols and recommendations for the patient's symptoms.

A patient defines the correct test as the one that uncovers the actual cause of the problem she is experiencing.

Notice the difference between the two perspectives.

Physicians want to do the right thing by providing the same best care that another excellent physician would provide, no matter how arbitrary that standard may be.

Patients want the right thing, period.

The first is couched in a context.

The second is absolute.

We all want to get to the bottom of any diagnosis, but we must start at the top --- with a blank slate. First, a person notices something wrong. She brings this concern to a physician's attention. In doing so, she becomes a patient. The concern isn't a diagnosis. Rather, it is the noticed effect of some yet unknown diagnosis.

For example, a urinary tract infection can cause burning during urination. Meningitis can cause a headache and neck stiffness. Pneumonia can cause a cough. Yet many diagnoses other than pneumonia can also cause a cough, and not every pneumonia will.

Alana lacked neither a good pediatrician, nor good parents. Importantly, no error had been committed, except in retrospect. The *ultimately* correct test hadn't been ordered because no symptom had yet indicated that it was the correct test. Had her femur not broken to expose her tumor to the correct tests, I trust that her physician and parents would have resumed pursuit of diagnostic tests. Their pause in the search for a diagnosis wouldn't have lasted because they hadn't yet explained her pain. As the persistent pain would have driven a broader and broader search for a diagnosis, eventually they would have arrived at a correct test.

A diagnosis can be easily missed even by expensive, technologically advanced imaging. A diagnosis can be missed by skilled and diligent physicians using those expensive tests, without their making any medical error.

In contrast, the auto mechanic can use a diagnostic computer that thinks through exactly the same plan from which the automobile is built. The computer's diagnostic complexities can match almost exactly to the complexities of problems that can arise.

Not so for the physician approaching a patient with a symptom or concern. The physician doesn't have the original plan for the human machine programmed perfectly into his mental diagnosis computer. The physician, instead, must guess well from the first conversation.

A Close Shave

I remember a patient from my third year of medical school. Every night Thomas, a retired financial planner, would develop high fevers, chills, and sweats, then feel better by morning. This cycle persisted for a couple of weeks. He called his internist. After a few days of outpatient work-up, his physician admitted him to the hospital for closer observation. Thomas had a mildly elevated heart rate, even when the fevers had broken during daylight hours; this further raised the level of concern.

On his first day in the hospital, we ordered a CT scan of his chest and abdomen, almost as a blind search for something abnormal.

Unexpectedly, the CT showed a large mass in his liver. This broached the possibility of a liver cancer. We ordered an MRI to better characterize the mass. Concern remained high even after we reviewed the MRI, the afternoon of the second day. We arranged a biopsy of the liver mass for his third hospital day. On day five, the result from this biopsy taught us that his liver mass wasn't cancerous and was certainly not the source of his fevers. It was a benign growth that had probably been present for years if not decades.

The five days of discussing his case with the team on daily morning and afternoon rounds taught me something about the search for a diagnosis. The more senior members of the team were never satisfied that the quest to sort out the liver mass would explain Thomas' fevers. Even if it revealed a cancer quite worthy of treatment, it left the search to explain his other symptoms unsatisfied. Something tangible to chase down wasn't enough.

Each day, I searched books and journals for case reports and obscure articles trying to pin the fevers and heart rate to the liver mass. They wouldn't stick.

The more experienced physicians knew that finding *something* didn't satisfy the search for *the* thing causing Thomas' full array of symptoms. They disciplined their thinking by the application of a principle borrowed from the physical sciences called "Occam's razor."

Attributed to William of Occam, a logician and Franciscan friar, the principle was recorded in his time as *Numquam ponenda est pluralitas sine necessitate.* [Plurality must never be proposed without necessity.][2] The principle prioritizes unifying and simple explanations over complex and multiplied explanations. The razor pares down complexity to simpler truth.

It is both more common and more intellectually satisfying to identify a single diagnosis that explains all of a patient's symptoms rather than two or three diagnoses each explaining some of the symptoms. Occam's razor encourages physicians to probe more deeply. We should dig out the root of a patient's symptoms rather than cover each symptom with a band-aid as if it were a disease itself.

Occam's razor can also get in our way.

We can be so certain that only one diagnosis exists that we stop looking after finding a first. Fortunately, symptoms and test results and diagnoses usually fit well together. Even when temporarily distracted by another problem, we remain incompletely satisfied in our search until we find the critical diagnosis that ties it all together. When we find ourselves head scratching in the struggle to explain all of the complaints by the thus-far-identified abnormality, we usually keep digging for the root.

The adherence of Thomas' more experienced physicians to Occam's razor kept them from believing that the liver mass held all the answers that Thomas needed. But Occam's razor didn't give them the correct answers, only the persistent lack of an answer.

After morning rounds on that fifth day, we returned to the drawing board. Having seen the liver mass trail come abruptly and definitively to an end, we decided to return to the very beginning.

This poor man, exhausted by his racing heart and high fevers, feeling poked and prodded and perplexed by test after test for the liver mass chose to sit up in bed for a scrawny, bespectacled medical student to examine him one more time from head to toe.

Almost nothing presented itself to my ears or eyes or finger tips. Doubting myself, thinking that I might just be grasping for anything, I hesitantly asked the resident who accompanied me, "Could this be a swollen lymph node? Here, feel this little bump on the side of his neck."

I felt a smooth, small lump, no bigger than the end of my pinky finger, bouncing in the tissues beneath my fingers' pressure on his skin.

The resident washed her hands and felt Thomas' neck on both sides simultaneously to compare.

"Maybe," she acknowledged. "Pretty subtle. Although I guess we have nothing else to go on. Let's get it biopsied."

A needle biopsy of this lymph node demonstrated a thyroid cancer, which could much more plausibly explain Thomas' fevers, weight loss, and elevated heart rate.

The correct diagnosis only followed our chasing down of an accidentally identified lymph node, barely palpable in his neck. Good thinking, such as that directed by Occam's razor, can protect us from some erroneous conclusions. Finding the correct ones, however, sometimes requires a little luck.

Seconds

George El-Khoury focuses his radiology practice on imaging of the musculoskeletal system. I had the privilege of spending a month with him during my internship at the beginning of orthopaedic surgical residency.

He had a gifted eye.

"Very interesting!" he would call out in his Lebanese accent from across the room.

Each time, at a glance from 15 feet, he had identified an unusual and intriguing finding or diagnosis on some film directly in front of me.

His glance beat my best attention every time.

Or he would walk into the room while I scrolled through the large panels of films on a light board. A radiograph only partway rolled over the light source would show enough that he would stop my scrolling and ask me to go back and look more carefully. Dr. El-Khoury's eyes rapidly identified findings.

But as talented as he was, he most *valued* diligence and discipline in radiology.

"Kevin, what is the most frequently missed diagnosis?" he asked at least two or three times each day during my month with him.

All of the radiology residents and fellows, accustomed to his question, would respond as a chorus: "The second diagnosis!"

"Satisfaction of search is the bane of the radiologist's existence,"

Dr. El-Khoury would explain. In his opinion, the specialty of radiology has little to do with talent. It has everything to do with discipline. Excellence derives from a regimented, thorough approach.

Dr. El-Khoury has organized studies of radiologists or other physicians who interpret radiographs. His studies measure the ability to decipher multiple findings on a single panel of images.

I participated in one of Dr. El-Khoury's studies as an orthopaedic resident, a few years after that month with him. By that point in training, I had grown comfortable with radiographs and scans of all varieties focused on the musculoskeletal system.

For the study, participant physicians reviewed all of the images from a series of trauma patients. Most patients had at least a CT scan of the neck and plain radiographs of the chest and pelvis. ER physicians obtain this cluster of images, called the "trauma series," on every victim of a high-energy accident, such as a car crash or fall from a roof. The study tested how well physicians looking at the images could identify all of the important injuries.

Throughout the hours sitting at the computer terminal as a study participant, my mind repeated his adage, "The most frequently missed diagnosis is the second diagnosis." Even knowing that finding second diagnoses was the entire point of the study, I found that it required incredible discipline not to stop looking at a study after identifying one abnormality. Certainly, most images in the study cases didn't have second findings, but some did. I would guess that more did than I correctly identified.

I never learned how well or poorly my interpretations compared to others in the study. It doesn't really matter. I'm not a radiologist. I may look at a lot of imaging myself, but I use imaging in a very different way. I *can* focus entirely on the first diagnosis because some radiologist with masterful self-discipline has already thoroughly reviewed the same images and ruled out the possibility of a second. Importantly, who reviews the diagnostic testing and by what discipline she reviews it will powerfully impact what she sees there.

I review images with the discipline of an orthopaedic surgeon. A radiologist reviews them with the discipline of a radiologist. We will not necessarily see the same diagnoses.

Cutthroat

Scars, scratches, and healing abrasions peppered Jackie's arms. A thick black leather biker's jacket hung on the side of her chair in the clinic room. Her face didn't match this toughness, though. Jackie looked worried. She hailed from an out-of-the-way small town, a few hours' drive from our cancer center. She arrived in my clinic by no direct route.

Jackie first called her family doctor about a lump just above the elbow, deep in the muscle. In retrospect, she thought that part of her arm had probably ached for a couple of weeks prior to her noticing the mass, but she had thought little of it. Bumps and bruises were standard fare in off-road motor biking.

Since noticing the lump, she was confident that it had steadily ached. It hurt less, though, than the back of her wrist and thumb. She could see nothing obviously wrong in the hand or wrist, but the skin prickled and burned with occasional lancing pains. When she saw her family doctor about the arm lump, he ordered an MRI. Her government program insurance refused an MRI for evaluation of the mass. It didn't refuse a referral to a neurosurgeon for the wrist pain that her physician felt was nerve-related.

Jackie asked the neurosurgeon about the mass in her arm, but he more or less rebuffed her. At least this is how she explained it to me. The neurosurgeon guessed that the pain in the wrist fit with nerve irritation from a slipped disc in the neck. Jackie insisted that her neck didn't hurt, but --- quite correctly --- the neurosurgeon explained that disc problems in the neck don't always cause pain in the neck itself. They more often cause pain somewhere in the arm, forearm, or hand, depending on the disc's level in the neck. Nursing attendants wheeled Jackie to the MRI scanner in the surgeon's office. The neck MRI identified a bulging disc; this was felt to be the culprit. The neurosurgeon scheduled surgery to remove the offending disc the next day.

Surgery added a horizontal scar to Jackie's throat. It also changed the previously conspicuous lack of neck pain: Jackie's neck hurt after surgery, but not beyond the reach of the pain pills provided by the surgeon. The burning pain in her wrist hadn't changed.

Between the time of her surgery and her follow-up appointment, two weeks later, the wrist and thumb pain had actually increased, as had the size of the arm mass. That the surgery didn't help her wrist pain frustrated Jackie, but less than her growing suspicion that the so-far-ignored arm mass might be cancer. The neurosurgeon sent her back to her family doctor.

This primary care physician called my office. I saw Jackie a couple of days after this call.

In my office, I noticed a large, smooth bump protruding from Jackie's arm as if she had an extra muscle just above the elbow. Muscle should be squishy, but this mass felt firm and stuck onto the bone underneath it.

I examined the muscle strength and skin sensation in her forearm and hand. She had poor strength in the muscles that should straighten the wrist and fingers. She felt little of my touching or even pricking the skin on the back of the thumb and wrist. She did say that touching that region increased the tingling she felt.

What had her surgeon been thinking?

He was a neurosurgeon, wasn't he?

Shouldn't that imply that he understood the anatomy of nerves?

He had focused attention on the spine in her neck because he felt the wrist pain came from irritation of the nerve exiting the spinal cord at the 6th level. The nerve at this level does give sensation to the skin on the back of the thumb and wrist. It also gives sensation to the palm side of the same region. It also drives the elbow-flexing power of the biceps muscle. Jackie had no problems on the palm and no weakness in her biceps muscle.

This imperfect fit between her symptoms and his diagnosis would be more than excusable if Jackie hadn't had a perfectly fitting diagnosis staring the surgeon in the face. Irritation of the radial nerve *will* cause tingling on only the back of the wrist and thumb, not the palm side. Irritation of the radial nerve *will not* weaken the biceps, but rather the muscles that extend the wrist and fingers. Irritation of the radial nerve arises not in the neck, but most frequently in the region of the arm where Jackie happened to have a large mass growing. *I* was irritated, to be sure.

Fortunately, the neurosurgeon had executed the spine surgery proficiently; no serious harm had been done. Further, I was able to explain to Jackie that rather than a delayed diagnosis of cancer, she had a benign mass that would resolve itself. I made this diagnosis by the characteristic appearance of her tumor on imaging. We had only to wait patiently for the inflammation within it to settle down. In fact, I planned to do nothing beyond waiting and re-imaging again in a few weeks.

Her immediate fear of cancer relieved, Jackie left my office quite happy. It pleased me to help protect her at least from any further unnecessary surgeries.

A little correct information as good as ended her frustration.

It only began mine.

I wanted to call the neurosurgeon. Was his jump to operate an honest mistake? Was he just diagnosing the neck problem because he had a solution for it?

Or was his decision financially driven?

I also wanted to call the government insurance program and rail against upside-down bureaucratic regulations that preferred to give a woman an unnecessary surgery rather than simply evaluate the real problem with the medically indicated MRI of her arm.

I did neither.

If her neurosurgeon made an honest mistake, he probably already knew it. At the very least, he would understand upon reading my letter how the correct diagnosis directly explained her nerve pain. As for the state insurance making spine surgery more accessible than an MRI of her arm, a phone call wouldn't change that.

Diagnosis through clinical examination can be challenging, I thought, in the nerves especially so. Perhaps Jackie didn't empha-size the arm mass as much to the neurosurgeon as she remembers doing. Perhaps the mass wasn't as visibly obvious two weeks prior when the neurosurgeon had decided to obtain a spine MRI and operate. Perhaps the subtle finger and wrist weakness, the primary means of differentiating between the two possible nerve sources of wrist pain was less prominent earlier in the course of the disease.

I wished I could see that neck MRI, to check in retrospect the severity of the disc problem for myself.

The MRI of a section of anyone's spine, as long as they are

over 20 years old, will frequently show degenerative abnormalities.[3] Nearly all of us have something torn, protruding, or inflamed from the effects of aging. That doesn't mean that we should all run out and get an MRI of the spine. Quite the contrary, it means that interpreting such abnormalities as problems requiring intervention can be extremely problematic.

We know one thing. Whatever abnormality was visible in Jackie's neck, it hadn't been causing any symptoms that its removal would resolve.

Why did the surgeon get the neck MRI in the first place?

Well, the scanner was sitting right there in his office. A disc problem *can* explain burning pain in the wrist. Maybe the arm mass was unrelated. Occam's razor would argue against this thinking, but he may have been thinking more about his own scalpel than Occam's razor.

It is so easy for physicians to jump to the ordering of any expensive diagnostic test. He might not have had much reason at all. Perhaps it was ordered when the patient was scheduled for the appointment. The governmental insurance program doesn't limit access to spine MRIs as it does to those for the arm.

When Jackie's surgeon ordered the MRI of her neck, the die was cast, to some extent. He held ready a cervical spine surgery. He only had to find a patient on whom to use it.

One of my professors in residency frequently joked that nothing is more dangerous than a surgeon with an open OR schedule and a mortgage to pay. That may not be fair to say at all in this situation, but even a well-intentioned surgeon looking at an MRI can find something in need of attention. Many patients want to hear nothing other than that a physician has a quick fix for their problem. If they have driven hours to get to the office, as Jackie had to see this neurosurgeon, the fix better be all the quicker.

As physicians or patients, when we *want* to find some specific diagnosis, we often will. A patient shopping among potential physicians will eventually find one who agrees with him. A physician looking hard enough for it can usually diagnose a problem that she knows how to treat. The uncertainty of diagnosis grants persuasive power to our wanting any specific diagnosis. Unfortunately, this wanting itself enhances the uncertainty in return.

Out of Context

For some diagnostic tests, we base the interpretation entirely on number thresholds. Computers can designate some lab values as high or low and even critically high or critically low. Of course, even these black-and-white lab test results must be applied to the patient's situation by a physician aware of the circumstance of the test.

Other tests, however, are not as black and white, even in the results themselves, let alone their application. I mentioned earlier that I review imaging with the discipline of an orthopaedic surgeon, not a radiologist. Part of the discipline I apply as an orthopaedic surgeon interpreting imaging is the context of a patient's history and physical examination findings. I can even go back and forth from the imaging on my computer screen to the examination room a few times, if necessary. In some clinics, I can pull the images up on a monitor in the patient's room.

Radiologists don't have this luxury. They depend on the history provided by the ordering physician. These days, they rarely, if ever, even see the patient directly. Radiologists instead read digital films at a remote, if not far distant, location.

I still smile when I remember one radiologist, who would melodramatically start to tremble when looking at imaging that demonstrated no clear abnormality.

As his chair rattling reached a fevered pitch, he would mutter, "I'm getting nervous. . . ."

Then again, louder, "I'm getting nervous. . . ."

Then louder still, "I'm getting nervous. . . ."

Finally, he'd burst out with, "Normal! I'll see you in court!"

His antics were intended to entertain only, but as with most humor, there was plenty of truth at its foundation. He knew that calling the result of a complex test such as an imaging study "normal" was a significant medico-legal and, more importantly, ethical responsibility. He understood that he rarely knew specifically why a physician had requested the imaging. He knew that he also lacked any meaningful historical details. He was left to the hard facts of the image itself.

This radiologist impressed upon me the need to record on an imaging requisition any helpful historical details or any specific question I was asking as an ordering physician --- details that are rarely provided by ordering physicians.

Some tests decidedly lack any such details, not simply by the laziness of the ordering physician, but by the tests' designed intention. Screening tests have the double-whammy of being tests without histories attached as well as tests with generally high stakes. Radiologists are usually most "nervous," for example, when reading screening mammography for this precise reason. Any disease prompting screening tests is a disease bearing significant impact on a person's health and well-being. We don't bother to screen for unimportant diseases.

For screening tests, the only requirement for the ordering of the test is the perception of risk. This might be age-, gender-, or exposure-related. There must be a high-risk group, for which iden-tification of disease before symptoms call attention to it can lead to more successful treatment outcomes than the usual treatment of symptom-identified disease.

Physicians measure the value of screening tests the same way they measure treatments. The provision of a certain screening test for a group of people is an intervention, the effect of which can be measured by outcomes. Because some screening tests have risks, one wants to be confident that the early identification of disease by screening provides more benefit than the potential problems induced by the screening itself.

Mammography provides an excellent example. As a screening test, mammography has been studied more thoroughly than any other. More than half a million women have enrolled in random-ized controlled trials of mammography. Three studies published in the 1980s "proved" the utility of routine screening mammography in the prevention of breast cancer deaths in specific populations.[4]

The entry criteria for each study have generated much controversy since. All three permitted enrollment of some women in their forties. Each woman enrolled in the experimental arm received yearly or biannual mammography. The studies continued for years. While the overall reduction in death from breast cancer in two of the studies wasn't significant, it was significant in the older portions of each of the groups studied.

What does that "prove?" Not a whole lot. This left a significant challenge to the medical community.

Should mammography be offered to women over forty, or only to those over fifty?

Beyond the cost and discomfort of mammography, there exists the real possibility that mammography might worsen outcomes in younger populations. Additional x-ray exposure in younger women could actually increase cancer risk. The false-negative mammography results, more readily obtained when imaging through younger breast tissue, might discourage other screening examinations that would be more effective at identifying cancers in the younger age group.

Of course, expert panels met, deliberated, and pontificated over the data, ultimately deciding in the United States that it would be wrong to withhold access to mammography from women in their forties. After all, more must be better, right? It's the American way. To this day there is little evidence that mammography saves the lives of women in their forties. Nonetheless, the recent suggestion that the recommendations ought to scale back to include only women above fifty was met with woeful, grandstanding speeches in the halls of Congress and elsewhere.

Politicians were scared to withhold the benefit of breast cancer screening by some regulation that permitted insurance companies or government health programs not to cover it. They *assumed* it was beneficial. They failed to recognize that a bigger question hadn't been answered.

No one questions the provision of clearly beneficial screening, but should we mandate screening for women of ages for which screening hasn't been shown to be beneficial?

That remains uncertain. Perhaps the uncertainty is less in need of political speeches and declarations and more in need of physicians being as honest as they can with themselves and their patients about what mammography can and cannot accomplish.

The failure of physicians to discuss mammography honestly with their patients has created a problem. Whether governments should insist that insurance carriers pay for mammography for women in their forties concerns me much less than the propaganda that has led women to trust this technology with all their hopes and fears.

Forget financial costs. Telling women that this test will keep them safe from age forty onward is simply not true by any way that we can actually measure.

Why have we encouraged them to believe it will?

Are we simply hoping that people will trust medicine more if they think we have more solutions to offer?

What if our solutions don't solve any problems?

Maybe we could try encouraging people to trust medicine by insisting on honesty instead.

Another screening test with different controversies inherent to it is colonoscopy. For colonoscopy as well, recommendations have been somewhat arbitrarily made. Like mammography, colonoscopy is uncomfortable and may or may not actually provide benefit from the identification of earlier-stage, more successfully treated pre-cancerous lesions.

Unlike screening mammography, however, colonoscopy is an invasive, expensive, and risky procedure. I personally know two men who were severely injured by colonoscopy, one a physician and the other a business executive. Each essentially lost a year of his life to critical medical care, multiple surgeries, and healing time. Each began this lost year from an intestinal tear during routine screening colonoscopy.

We cannot judge the risks of the procedure by these stories. That isn't fair. Obviously, the rates of complications such as these are extremely low. The rates are not zero, however. So risks have to be balanced against any real benefit in deaths prevented from colon cancer.

Colon cancer --- perhaps more than any other cancer whose biology has been studied --- follows a fairly rigid sequence of events in the progression from a polyp into a high-grade, deadly cancer. We quite prefer plucking out a polyp to the interventions required when full-blown colon cancer has set in.

So how often is frequent enough to screen?

The interval for recommended screening colonoscopy has ranged from as low as yearly to as high as once each decade after age fifty. Recently, it has landed in between these. What is interesting to our discussion here is that whatever the recommended interval, it will determine how the results must be interpreted. If a patient is going to have another screening colonoscopy a year later, an early-appearing polyp might be safely noted and checked again in a year. If the next screening colonoscopy will not happen for another decade, that polyp (despite the fact that most like it would never become dangerous) might just have to be removed on first sighting.

Because tests are interpreted, context matters immensely. Physicians responsible for interpreting screening tests receive few contextual medical clues to aid in that interpretation. Each society creates the critical context of any screening test by deciding who will be screened and how often. Only the population that policy, propaganda or insurance programs determine to be "at risk" will have access to the uncertainties that transpire once the tests are undertaken.

Horse Tale

Anne Osborne has been said by some to have literally written the book on neuroradiology, the specialty focused on reviewing imaging of the brain and spinal cord. Dr. Osborne's career has spanned the development of neuroradiology, which really came into its own as complex three-dimensional imaging technologies became available. I have heard her joke, "Hey, I am really good, as long as I have about 15 million dollars of equipment available." Most of her work involves the interpretation of very expensive-to-obtain tests.

Dr. Osborne remembers when her university hospital installed its first MRI scanner in the early 1980s. "Everyone was excited for the capacity to image the human brain without radiation. The only problem was that we had no idea what normal actually looked like."

She had a friend down the street from where she had lived at that time who was a little over 100 years old. Excited for the opportunity to be perhaps the first to see the centenarian brain by MRI and knowing that no significant risk was involved, Dr. Osborne asked her friend if he would agree to a brain scan. His response showed the wisdom of his ten decades of life.

"Annie, I don't think that would be a good idea. You see, I am happy, fairly healthy, and have no head problems at the moment. If you look in my brain, you might just find a problem. Honestly, at my age, I would rather not know what you might find in there."

Not everyone demonstrates such wisdom. Dr. Osborne recalls the clamoring after total-body screening CT scans when that technology became available and the similar thronging for total body MRI that still persists today.

"What do you do *when* you find something?" she asks.

Dr. Osborne related one story that is apparently well known in the world of radiology. The chairman of a radiology department at a major university health center decided to enroll in a study after a scanner was installed at his institution. He got a CT scan of his own chest; not surprisingly, the scan wasn't entirely "normal."

It identified a mass in one of his lungs. A series of additional radiologic and eventually invasive diagnostic tests followed. Three months after the "screening" CT scan, the mass was confirmed to be nothing more than residual scar-like tissue from a prior infection.

"Not all of this technology is available to patients as readily as it was available to that Radiology Department chairman." Dr. Osborne reminded me. "No. We do have our standards! In the middle of the night and on weekends, we limit access to advanced imaging. MRI technicians are no happier about crawling out of bed at 2 AM to man the scanner than you or I would be. I am the one who will have to call them to come in from home and scan.

"Obviously, as the radiologist on call, I am happy to phone in the troops for a patient in need, but I try to be sure that there is an actual patient who is actually in need. I'd rather not call them in for a physician simply in need of the convenient availability of the test."

The most common request for after-hours neurologically-related

MRIs comes documented as "rule-out *cauda equina* syndrome." *Cauda equina*, translated from Latin, means "horse tail."

This is, like many Latin anatomic terms, merely descriptive. The cauda equina is the large bundle of spinal nerve roots traveling down the spinal canal from the end of the spinal cord itself in the mid-back. These nerve roots supply all of the lower extremity sensation and muscles, as well as the anal and bladder sphincters.

Their sudden dysfunction, called cauda equina syndrome, usually results from physical compression of the nerve roots by a slipped disc, tumor or fracture. Unlike spinal cord tissue, these nerve roots maintain some regenerative potential. This means that the cauda equina can "take a joke" --- or at least recover after a mild jab. There are limits to the hits from which it can recover, but lost function in the cauda equina doesn't necessarily mean permanently lost function.

This inspires hope but also demands urgency in the correction of compression injury to the cauda equina. Symptoms may improve if the pressure can be released. The horse --- pun intended --- may not yet be out of the barn.

MRI is an excellent diagnostic test for cauda equina syndrome. The compression is usually readily visible. However, this expensive diagnostic test should follow the taking of a detailed history and the performance of a few, very simple physical examination maneuvers. Cauda equina syndrome isn't common. Nevertheless, the complaints and physical findings that suggest it as a diagnosis are not subtle. They are familiar to the emergency room physicians and spine specialists who order these MRIs.

They are also familiar to some patients. Some back pain patients have learned that complaining of bowel or bladder problems will prompt more attention in the ER. ER physicians or the spine specialists they consult may simply want MRIs in these patients to cover themselves medico-legally. No matter who might want this MRI, if it is after hours, the physician must contact the radiologist on-call to order it.

"Well, Kevin," Dr. Osborne continued, "I got just one page too many from a resident in the middle of the night. I asked him about the findings on the rectal examination. When he hesitated,

I refused to call in the technicians. I told him that I would call them only after he could phone me back with the specific rectal examination findings. He never called me back that night. I guess he hadn't really suspected cauda equina syndrome. Nonetheless, it got me thinking. I looked up all the emergent MRI consults for cauda equina syndrome for an entire year."

"How many really had it?" I asked, uncomfortably remembering the many 2 AM ER consults during my orthopaedics residency to come and clinically rule out cauda equina syndrome. I had performed a number of rectal examinations. I had even ordered a few MRIs. But I hadn't seen real cauda equina syndrome once in that setting.

"Oh, there were more than none, but not many more," she answered, dryly. "Almost all of the true positives had metastatic cancer to the spine or some obvious risk factor."

"And what about the rest?" I asked.

"Complete fakes," she answered tersely. "Not only did imaging confirm the absence of findings consistent with cauda equina syndrome, but review of the records showed that most had never even been properly examined in the first place.

"After completing this study, I had my guard up. Now I had data to hurl at anyone calling me inappropriately. Then, the last time I was on-call, just a couple of weeks ago, I got a cauda equina page from an ER resident. I drilled down on the history and physical examination findings. He stammered something about only having made the call on behalf of his attending. The attending called me back a few minutes later. It happened to be the chairman of the Division of Emergency Medicine. 'Anne,' he said, 'I put my finger in the rectum myself. This one is real. Please call in your team.' So I did!"

Not all technology can or should be available all of the time, awaiting only the whim of an ordering physician. Physicians struggle to decide when a given test is warranted or appropriate and what question it might answer. That decision must begin with honesty about what technology can and cannot accomplish. It must acknowledge the limits of diagnostic tests and couch those diagnostic tests in a firm framework of history and physical examination findings.

Access to advanced (read "expensive") diagnostic technologies practically defines American healthcare. This may no longer include MRIs in the middle of the night for the trumped-up suspicion of cauda equina syndrome when Dr. Osborne is on-call. Nonetheless we still order many expensive tests with almost reckless abandon. Our system only reimburses care providers for providing services; patients always want the latest and greatest technologies; neither directly pays for the cost of such technologies; and a physician feels threatened with serious liability if he fails to order such technologies when another physician might have.

Technologies and access to them naturally proliferate from all these factors. Having spent some of my training time in Canada, I am familiar with the challenges wrought by poorer access to these technologies. Limited access to imaging can delay diagnosis sometimes and frustrate or inconvenience patients at most times.

I don't advocate here for or against access to imaging or one kind of medical system over another. The problem of uncertainty taints every decision in every kind of system. When that uncertainty is exploited by bureaucrats trying to save a buck, clinicians trying to make a buck, or patients who are simply awed by impressive technologies, we start to seek additional testing. We seek it with the occasionally false hope that more test results will actually reduce uncertainty for our health; they might do nothing of the sort.

You have seen how uncertainty in diagnosis stubbornly persists even after physicians have ordered MRIs and CTs. Even when physicians apply careful discipline to avoid shallow partial diagnoses, or avoid missing second diagnoses, the correct diagnosis can yet remain elusive. Finding the correct diagnosis may require a classmate to kick your thigh during dance class or a medical student to wonder out loud if a tiny lump might be worth pursuing.

We must tread toward a diagnosis circumspectly, watching for any clues along the way --- and we must not forget that these clues don't necessarily come from more tests. You have seen tests lead to unnecessary additional tests as well as to unnecessary surgeries. Because diagnostic tests create new uncertainties as we order them, the context of their ordering and the decision to order them are most critical to guess correctly.

We will not always find out when we "get in there."

Starting Your Conversation. . . .

Impenetrable

Principle: There are no ultra-secret truths about diagnosis available beneath the skin for most conditions.

Ask your physician: What do you anticipate learning during the procedure that you don't already know about my condition?

Near Miss

Principle: Diagnosis can be fleeting. We can miss it entirely without committing any real error.

Ask your physician: If we were to broaden our search, what would you look for next?

A Close Shave

Principle: Occam's razor, or the preference for a single unifying diagnosis, keeps physicians looking for a root cause.

Ask your physician: How might my very different symptoms derive from one central problem?

Seconds

Principle: A physician's commitment to finding a single unifying diagnosis can get in her way if she stops looking after finding a first diagnosis.

Ask your physician: Are there any other findings or abnormalities uncovered by these tests that don't relate to my central problem? Do they require any follow-up at a later time, after we have finished with our current focus?

Cutthroat

Principle: Physicians and patients have to check themselves or they will too easily find what they want to find.

Ask your physician: What diagnosis do you personally hope to find in the results of my test? What do you think that I want you to find in the results?

Out of Context

Principle: Tests are most informative when they are ordered with specific questions in mind. Screening tests usually are ordered with only general questions in mind.

Ask your physician: What question will the result of this test answer for you about my condition? If there is no specific question, have people in my own situation been tested and found to benefit from this screening?

Horse Tale

Principle: Access to tests, determined by health systems, can change what those tests mean when they are performed.

Ask your physician: To what diagnostic test do you wish I had access? Would you be disappointed if our system didn't permit me to get this test, or is this beyond what is really critical?

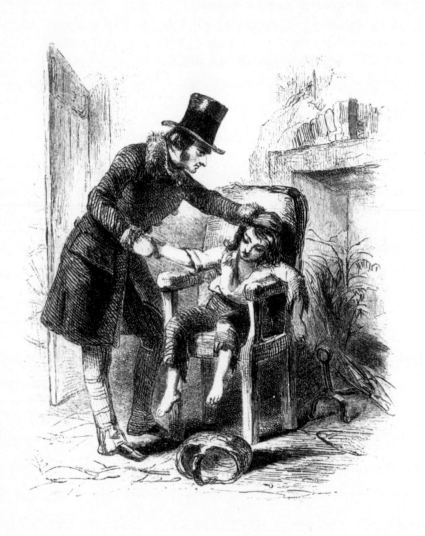

TESTING TESTS

Positive Results

"Thanks for seeing her. She is a serious athlete for a 12-year-old, but I'm confident that she has no sports-related problem in her knee," the referring orthopaedic surgeon told me.

He called me in the early evening of a Friday, after seeing Lilly in his office for knee pain. Radiographs obtained upon her arrival there had shown a tumor in the fibular head, a bone structure just below the knee.

I reviewed the radiographs he had sent electronically, then arranged some additional imaging, as well as a biopsy of the mass. I met Lilly when she came in a couple of days later for the biopsy. I had spoken with her mother by phone a few times, but as I had been focusing primarily on the imaging studies and the challenges of arranging additional tests on the weekend, I hadn't yet had the chance to get the full story.

Lilly was indeed a serious athlete. She played outdoor soccer in the spring, summer and fall, then indoor soccer in the winter, including both a local and a travel team each season. Accustomed to minor aches and pains, she had ignored the knee pain for a couple of months until it really began to impede her play. It also troubled her sleep at night. Initially mild swelling in the knee had worsened slowly, never responding to her usual solution: rest, ice and elevation.

Ten days before going to see the sports surgeon, she visited her pediatrician's office to have her knee pain evaluated. The pediatrician, who knew Lilly well, noticed that she looked tired and maybe a little weak. According to Lilly's mother, the pediatrician was concerned that Lilly might be sicker than just having a knee problem. With the mild general systemic illness as her backdrop, the pediatrician performed a rapid strep test swab. This was positive. She then started Lilly on an antibiotic.

Although the diagnosis of strep throat in the absence of soreness in the throat perplexed them, Lilly and her mother followed the instructions dutifully. When nothing improved within a week, they made the sports clinic appointment, assuming that the knee pain and the strep throat were totally unrelated.

Lilly finished her course of antibiotics the day she saw me. We didn't discuss in detail what it had accomplished for her. I doubt that Lilly ever had an asymptomatic strep throat but will never know for certain. I was quite impressed that the pediatrician had noted the mild general tiredness and weakness of which Lilly hadn't complained. I agreed that (even after the antibiotics) she was slightly blunted in her energy level from what I would expect in a girl accustomed to the rigors of her athletic schedule.

The type of cancer that I found in Lilly's leg can cause symptoms suggestive of an infection. It is rare enough that I wouldn't expect any general pediatrician to think of it before deciding she had a strep throat and a sports injury.

A strep throat infection that persists long enough *can* cause mild systemic symptoms and even an inflamed knee. The pediatrician linked all these possibilities together. She ordered a test.[1] The positive result confirmed her suspicion.

Lilly must have had strep throat, right?

Well, she *might* have.

Alternatively, the result may have been a false-positive. False-positives and false-negatives happen with every diagnostic test. Unable to erase this fundamental uncertainty in diagnosis, physicians instead strive to *manage* it by understanding each test. Physicians characterize tests by sensitivity, or the tendency to avoid false-negatives, and specificity, the tendency to avoid false-positives.

Lilly's pediatrician probably ordered the rapid strep test because it is a rather specific test. Unfortunately, even relatively specific tests can still have false-positives.

As you might guess, sensitivity and specificity compete with each other. Consider the test of a pulse rate as an example. Physicians arbitrarily set the definition of an abnormally fast pulse at 100 beats per minute. Not every positive result poses a danger. The diagnosis of an abnormally fast heart rate demands an explanation, but that may be as simple as, "Doc, I just ran up the stairs to avoid being late for my appointment."

Heart rates vary widely between different people. A heart rate of 80 for a serious endurance athlete might be abnormally fast, but would be called negative or normal by our test result. If we were to lower the definition of abnormal to 80, we would reduce such false-negatives. However, that lower threshold would increase false-positives, as we call the normal resting heart rate of many less athletic individuals "abnormal." It would increase sensitivity in exchange for decreased specificity.

Physicians talk about these as bell curve distributions. There is a distribution of normal and a distribution of abnormal, with lots of overlap between the two.

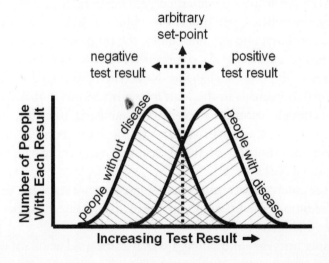

Physicians and patients would love to widen the gap between the normal and abnormal bell curves. This would permit increased sensitivity and specificity. Unfortunately, very few tests do this. The width of each bell curve and the overlap of the abnormal and normal bell curves principally reflect the fuzzy uncertainty in any biological system.

Heaping uncertainty on top of this fuzziness is the fact that we can only measure the sensitivity and specificity of a given test if we have a background definition of *truth* for comparison. Testing tests requires knowing the correct answer in the end.

In Lilly's case, no one will ever know if she really had strep throat or not.

Standards & Poor

Tests are tested against established gold standard diagnoses. By "established" I mean decided or determined. Gold standard diagnostic truth is rarely apparent by simple observation. If it were, we wouldn't need diagnostic tests at all.

The definition of a gold standard diagnosis can change over time. As technology improves, some new advances are significant enough to change the very definition of a disease.

Marfan syndrome, an inherited genetic disease, provides one excellent example. Once defined by clinical features, such as tall stature and heart and eye difficulties, the diagnosis was made by *adding up* these features.[2] As clinicians recognized new features of the disease, the criteria changed. New criteria managed to lump additional individuals in the Marfan syndrome group that hadn't shown enough features to meet prior standards. Recently, some children of individuals with Marfan syndrome have been diagnosed before manifesting any of the clinical features, simply by genetic tests from a cheek swab.

As the criteria have changed over time, the gold standard, or the very definition of who does and doesn't have Marfan syndrome, has also changed.

During my years in training, I watched the gold standard diagnostic definitions change for many of the diseases I treat in practice.

Return with me to Lilly's story. Our discussion of her strep-throat conundrum didn't bring us to the end of the uncertainty in her diagnosis. I noted that the cancer type I "found" in Lilly's leg offered an alternate explanation for her generally ill feeling.

How did I really *find* that diagnosis?

First, I reviewed the radiographs of her knee. As the tumor had grown through Lilly's fibula, the bone had tried to react and wall off its progress, failing each time. This growth pattern left a layered look to the surface of the bone. We call it "onion skinning." The onion skinning on Lilly's fibula led us to suspect a tumor called Ewing's sarcoma, the second most common bone cancer in children.

With an expectation of finding Ewing's sarcoma, I performed a biopsy next. For Ewing's sarcoma in particular, the analysis of biopsies has changed dramatically across the last two decades.[3] The way that Ewing's sarcoma was originally defined was by the appearance of a shaving of biopsy tissue under a microscope using standard dyes called H&E. No one ever trusted this standard as being all that golden since Ewing's sarcoma cells look like those of many other tumors, round and dark blue on H&E. Lymphomas, in particular, can look the same, but should be treated quite differently.

The pathologist called me a couple of days after Lilly's biopsy with no good news to report.

"You've got to be kidding me!" I responded in disbelief. "You couldn't find any living cells in the three grams of tissue I submitted?" I learned that most of the tumor cells in the processed specimen showed only the ghostly shadows of dead cells, a problem frequent for Ewing's sarcoma, but also common among lymphomas. So the original standard for diagnosis wasn't going to help us.

About 1990, pathologists learned that Ewing's sarcoma cells on slides will light up with a special antibody dye called CD99. This typically adds an additional day to the diagnostic process, but quickly replaced the use of H&E dyes as the gold standard definition of disease.

The pathologist offered, "I'll see if I can pick up any cells staining positively for CD99. It's unlikely, but worth a try."

I agreed. "The story and radiographic findings are so classic that we need no more than a hint toward Ewing's to confirm this, but we have to have a hint. Maybe some of the dead cells will take up the stain."

The next afternoon the pathologist called me back.

The cells hadn't stained with CD99.

Two strikes.

By the end of the 1990s, scientists had realized that almost every Ewing's sarcoma has a specific gene alteration, called a transloca- tion. Pathologists began using tests for the translocation as an extra confirmation of Ewing's sarcoma in the early 2000s. They initially tested the sensitivity and specificity of the translocation tests against the gold standard of CD99, but then began to think that the translocation tests trumped CD99.

The gold standard changed again.

"What about molecular testing?" I suggested. "We don't need living cells for molecular testing."

"Okay, we'll run the molecular tests," the pathologist said. "But you should get Lilly scheduled to come in for another biopsy just in case."

I reluctantly scheduled Lilly for a second surgical biopsy.

The first round of molecular tests failed to identify the most common Ewing's sarcoma translocation in Lilly's tumor sample. An alternate translocation (present in less than 10 percent of cases) was found the next morning.

An hour later, I met Lilly and her mother in the pre-operative area of the hospital. Rather than checking her in for a repeat biopsy as planned, I walked them up to the chemotherapy unit. Lilly would get treatment for a diagnosis made by application of a new diagnostic standard --- not a new standard confirming what an old standard already told us, but a new standard standing alone by itself.

On some fundamental level, even gold standards for diagnosis are fluid. Before we can begin treating a problem, our process of diagnosis must lump entities with like entities and split between entities that behave differently or are treated differently. In Lilly's case, we needed a nudge toward lumping it with a typical Ewing's sarcoma or a nudge toward splitting it from an unusual lymphoma.

No matter how golden or how standard, the molecular test happily obliged with both needed nudges.

Agreeing upon standard criteria for diagnosing any specific disease is one way that physicians manage the uncertainty of diagnosis. Not surprisingly, new uncertainties arise as these criteria change over time. As diagnostic gold standards evolve, they change the cases included in each disease-specific group. Do we know that Ewing's sarcoma defined by the molecular test will behave the same way as Ewing's sarcoma defined by CD99? Do we know that it will respond to the same treatments? Of course not. We can expect large overlaps between the two groups, as many tumors would have been called Ewing's sarcoma by either definition, but overlaps, as you saw in the bell-curves, make for rather imprecise knowledge.

Competing Catechisms

"Always be dogmatic!" Dr. Unni slapped glass slides from a stack of consult cases onto the microscope platform in front of him. He didn't even take his eyes from the scope. He flashed through slides and cases, blurting the diagnosis for each to his pathology fellow, who feverishly scribbled notes onto a pile of papers.

"I tell my fellows: Always be dogmatic," he repeated, never slowing his march through the stack of cases.

A handful of seconds was all any single slide received of his attention. "Look at this one," he said, pausing on one slide. "What do you see?" He leaned to the side and motioned for me to look into the eyepieces over his shoulder.

"There are blood-filled spaces with intervening stromal background," I began. "I see a lot of giant cells and some scant benign-appearing woven bone."

"Nobody cares for you to *describe* what you see. What *is* it?"

"Is it an aneurysmal bone cyst?" I offered hesitantly.

"Wrong!" After pausing a moment, he stated more emphatically, "It *is* an aneurysmal bone cyst!" and took over the eyepieces again. As he reached for the next case, he muttered, "Always be dogmatic. . . ."

Krishnan K. Unni is one of the most prominent bone tumor pathologists of the twentieth century; some would argue that only Dr. David C. Dahlin, his mentor and teacher, overshadows him. Between the two of them, they interpreted all of the bone tumor cases at the Mayo Clinic for half a century.

On this occasion, I was visiting the clinic for a job interview with the orthopaedic surgery department, full of its own giants in their respective fields. I was especially delighted to have Dr. Unni as one of my interviewers. He told me that he was already partly retired and would be fully retired before my proposed position would start.

"But until I finish, I read all these cases, every day." He motioned to the stack of reports and slide folders held by his fellow. "Luckily, when you've read the thousands of cases I've read, most don't take very long."

"How can you be sure so quickly?" I asked.

"Because I *am* the gold-standard," he replied.

I understood what he meant by this. Other skilled pathologists send him cases from around the world. Even if he renders no more than his opinion, it is the opinion of one of the most experienced and recognized in the field. I didn't get the impression that he was trying to be arrogant at all. He was simply stating a fact.

"But don't you have to explain in your report why you think a certain case is a certain diagnosis?"

"No. I often delete half of the descriptive text the fellows dictate in the note. Long pathology reports are wishy-washy. I want the referring pathologist or surgeon to know precisely what I think the lesion is. As a pathologist, if I always hedge and describe, I might never be wrong, but I will also never be right. It is exactly why I always tell my fellows to be dogmatic. Come down on a diagnosis!"

How will anyone ever know if Dr. Unni is right or wrong? As inspiring as his confidence may be, it can only really work for diagnoses that have no other, more objective gold standard. For such diagnoses, we cannot measure the sensitivity or specificity of his opinion as a diagnostic test. We can compare Dr. Unni's opinion to the opinions of other experienced and famous referral bone pathologists, his peers.

I had the rare opportunity to do this once.

The comparison didn't offer sensitivity and specificity as outputs, but measured how consistent his opinion was with his peers for making a certain diagnosis. In other words, how much was the diagnosis for a given case an apparent fact, visible to any expert, versus an arbitrary judgment made by each? I mentioned that K. K. Unni was one of the most prominent bone pathologists, but he isn't alone at the top of the bone pathology prominence pyramid. There are a few others in his league.

I remember a brief conversation with one of these other bone pathology experts, Andrew Rosenberg, who then worked at Massachusetts General Hospital. When I called to ask him to participate in my comparison study, he responded, "Of course I'll participate. In return, you have to call me when all the data is in to let me know which ones my colleagues got wrong!"

By all reports, Dr. Rosenberg charges at his work with the same competitive drive and spirit that I heard through the phone line. Medical students and residents alike who have worked with him describe wide-eyed witnesses of Dr. Rosenberg attacking massive bone tumor specimens with the band saw. Pathologists in many centers relegate the process of dividing specimens into manageably-sized pieces to technicians or trainees, but not Dr. Rosenberg. His enthusiasm spilled over on the phone, rapidly dismissing my thanks for his participation in our study. I could not see, but I imagined that his hands were gesticulating wildly while he spoke.

The study compared the pathologists' interpretations of imaging and glass slides from a mixed group of cartilage tumors in bones.[4] The tumors included highly aggressive cancers and some growths so inactive that I cannot even appropriately apply the term "tumor" to them. The pathologists were to sort them into finite groups of benign, low-grade cancerous, and high-grade cancerous lesions.

Our results basically showed poor agreement among the pathologists in this sorting procedure. These expert opinion gold standard diagnoses didn't agree with one another. The sad conclusion was that our best definitions for the diagnoses in this particular disease spectrum are not satisfactory. The distinctions between the three different groups appeared to be no more than arbitrary for some of the cases in the study. Beyond pathologic grading, no other better standard exists for comparison, especially when the grading judgment is passed down by pathologists of the likes of Andrew Rosenberg, K. K. Unni, or other members of this group.

While these experts appreciate that their opinions become the gold standard for each case in which they are involved, they also understand the limits in their discernment, perhaps even more so after completing the study. While Andrew Rosenberg delighted in the slightly competitive game that the study offered for sparring with his peers, he also recognizes that when he interprets real cases attached to real patients, it isn't a game; a surgeon will use his opinion to generate a treatment plan with real effects.

In some medical centers, surgeons will treat what their pathologist calls a low-grade chondrosarcoma (cartilage cancer) with radical surgery to remove an entire block of bone containing the mass. A reconstruction of the defect with large metal implants will follow this resection. The surgery has high risks in both the short-term and long-term. The implants can wear out or become infected even years after surgery.

An enchondroma, on the other hand, or benign cartilage growth, if scraped out of a bone usually leaves the surgeon feeling silly that she did a surgery on it at all. Most can and should be observed without intervention. As drastically disparate as these two treatment strategies are, you can see why both physicians and patients want to get the correct diagnosis in the first place. Unfortunately, this study showed that we may not be as good at making those diagnoses as we had hoped. We are, at least, not as consistent among different expert pathologists as we would hope to be.

When a dogmatic dictum sent down from an internationally recognized expert is the best standard we have, it is rather disconcerting to learn that the dictum will be different depending on which internationally recognized expert you happen to have asked. My coauthors and I managed this particular uncertainty in the diagnosis of cartilage tumors by exposing it to other physicians and publishing our results in the medical literature. But what next? Can we do better? Will we tell our patients how poorly we currently do?

Thorned Roses

A young man named Jason came to the orthopaedics clinic with an unusual problem. I was a resident at the time. His story began more than 10 years prior to our meeting. During his childhood, a thorn had pricked the front of his knee. Over a few days, the knee had grown swollen and red, prompting a surgery to drain infection from it. He had also been given antibiotics, he remembers, as an inpatient in the hospital for weeks. Eventually, the inflammation quieted down. Every year or two since, he had had an episode of severe knee pain and swelling that would then resolve over a few days. He had begun such an episode a week prior to coming to see me.

At first glance, his knee looked quite swollen, but I could feel no fluid within it. Instead, the patella, or knee cap, was expanded to about two and a half times its natural size in every dimension. Imaging of the knee confirmed this. It also suggested that the bone in the patella had more mineral than is typical. With its appearance, connected to his history, I explained to Jason that his patella was probably infected, and had been for years. I also explained that we can rarely, if ever, fully clear chronic infections from bones without removing the entire bone itself. Some chronic infections become latent or inactive as they are walled off inside a bone and may not cause problems for years at a time, but they don't resolve entirely.

Jason decided he wanted our team to biopsy his knee cap to see if we could find what bug was infecting it. I explained that I thought that he should consider biopsy primarily as a preamble to removal of the infected bone; biopsy alone posed a real risk of stirring up the long-quiet infection. He understood this risk. He wanted to get to the bottom of his mysteriously swollen knee. We scheduled the biopsy.

Cultures obtained from the bone didn't grow any bacteria, fungus, or tuberculosis. Pathology confirmed that microscopically, the bone appeared to have a chronic infection. To my surprise, Jason had no problems immediately after the biopsy. No infections stirred up.

Healing tissue had sealed over Jason's wound when he came to the clinic for a three-week follow-up appointment. He had experienced no fevers or chills or any local swelling in the knee itself. We reviewed the test results, the negative culture and positive pathology. I explained many possible reasons for the culture result being negative. The infection may have been so long dormant that no active bugs were present. None of the seven culture swabs I had obtained from the bone had grown any bacteria or fungus.

Jason decided to hold at that point and wait to see what happened. He knew that he might have a sudden flare of the infection at any time but was feeling reluctant about more surgery. He scheduled an appointment to check in with us in three months.

Three weeks later, I was the resident on-call when a page came from the emergency room. Jason had come there with questions. Well, far more than just questions --- Jason had a knee filled inside and out with pus. We had to take him urgently to the operating room. This time, with a very active infection, a bug grew from the cultures. The particular bacterium, called *pseudomonas*, fit well with his story of a thorn-prick as the initial source of the infection a decade earlier. We washed his knee out again two days later and removed the entire bone of his chronically infected knee cap. After a short course of antibiotics, Jason's knee was cleared of the infection, likely permanently.

Jason decided not to act on test results that informed us that his bone bore the signs of a chronic infection. He decided to believe another test result that failed to identify a specific bug as the cause of that infection. It's quite conceivable, especially with an entirely quiet knee three weeks following a surgical biopsy, that he might have continued on his prior course of a few days of irritation in the knee every year or two, but otherwise gotten along fairly well. Had we proceeded to remove his bone immediately after the mixed-result biopsy, we certainly would never have known that we had prevented the acute infection that ultimately transpired; we only would have lowered the *chance* for such an infection.

Jason's decision not to remove the patella initially can really be called the wrong decision only in retrospect. His experience from that point could have gone in either direction. Only when he suddenly developed a severely infected knee six weeks after the biopsy did we *know* which of the tests had been correct.

Jason's case models well the real test of tests: elapsed time. Better than comparing the result of one test to the results of another accepted standard test, or comparing one expert's opinion to that of another, observation of a disease's course over time is the ultimate gold standard for diagnosis. Especially if it is important, the diagnostic truth will usually become more --- not less --- clear as time passes.

Compartmentalizing

The batter returned Stephanie's neatly arching slow pitch as a line drive directly at her. She managed to catch it, but only after it smacked into her throwing arm just below the elbow. The out ending the inning. Stephanie won the junior varsity softball game.

"It was a good thing, too," Stephanie thought. She doubted she could possibly throw another pitch. There was nothing soft about the ball's contact with her flesh.

By the end of the pizza lunch she enjoyed with her parents and brother after the game, she began to think something must really be wrong. The forearm throbbed painfully. Her family changed afternoon plans and came straight to the emergency room from the pizza place.

Radiographs showed no broken bones, but the ER physician was sufficiently concerned to call the orthopaedics team.

The resident on call with me was filling out paperwork, preparing for our next surgery in the operating room. Saturdays can be busy at the children's hospital. He left to go check Stephanie's forearm when the page came for him. He returned a few minutes later to report Stephanie's story and his findings on physical examination. By that time, I was painting aseptic solution on a younger child's broken elbow, preparing to pin a break.

"I don't know," he confessed. "I'm worried she might be developing compartment syndrome."

Compartment syndrome is a challenging --- but critically important --- diagnosis to make. Compartments are body spaces defined at their borders by tough lining tissues. Like nylon jacket material, these linings don't stretch, even when the muscles within the compartments swell. Because the lining cannot expand, swelling raises the pressure within the compartment. Eventually, this increased pressure prevents blood flow within the small vessels. Poor blood flow depletes oxygen levels, further damaging the muscle and creating additional swelling, additional pressure.

If the pressure stays high enough for long enough --- and a few hours will suffice --- muscles, nerves, and vessels begin to die in earnest. By this point in its course, the diagnosis of compartment syndrome is blatantly obvious. Time has provided an unassailable gold standard for diagnosis. Unfortunately, we have no good treatments for compartment syndrome this far along.

"Well, this pinning will only take a few minutes," I replied. "Get scrubbed and help me here. Then we'll check Stephanie together."

Twenty minutes and three pins later, the resident and I removed our surgical gowns and headed back down to the ER. Even with some morphine now provided through an IV, Stephanie's pain had worsened. A round, purple bruise was ripening on the upper half of her forearm. The muscles beneath this were firm to touch, almost hard. I gently flexed and extended her index finger to stretch her forearm muscles without touching them directly. She grimaced.

A few minutes later Stephanie was rolling into the operating room.

Every time a surgeon correctly identifies compartment syndrome early in its course and reverses it, he averts disaster. Long incisions along the forearm will open the linings of each of the compartments. The swollen muscles within will burst with the release of pressure. We leave the long compartment release incisions open to keep the pressure from rebuilding. Long open incisions generate other problems: infections, the need for later skin grafts to cover the bulged-out muscles, and unsightly scars.

As frustrating as these treatment-induced challenges may be, they are quite happily exchanged for the horrific results of untreated compartment syndrome with its dead nerves, muscles, and vessels. On the other hand, treatment outcomes experienced from compartment releases performed when full-blown compartment syndrome wasn't in development are far from desirable. That said, once I decided to take Stephanie to the operating room to release

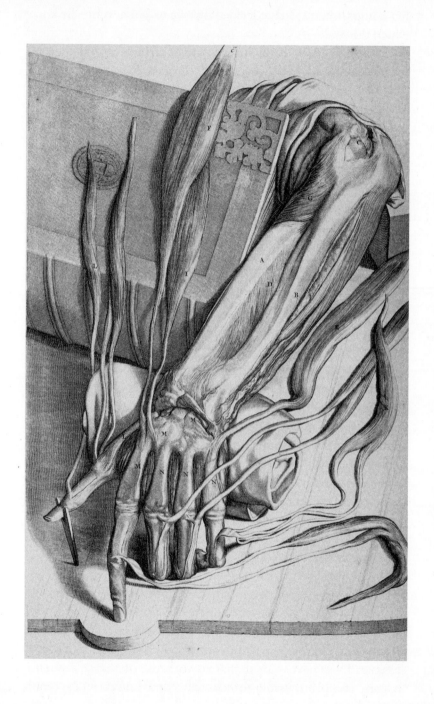

her compartments, I also decided that we would never really know which this was.

Compartment releases offer no final answer of whether the diagnosis was correctly made. They stop the course of disease that might later offer gold standard confirmation of the diagnosis.

Keeping the Faith

John Cameron was the chief of general surgery at Johns Hopkins Hospital for 19 years. Everything about the man screamed precision and control. From the narrow ties he wore tightly knotted between heavily starched, razor sharp collars to the shortly cropped hair that would have passed boot camp muster but never appeared to get long enough to require a fresh cut, the very look of him made you want to stand at attention. He had an almost spooky, all-knowing way about him. He seemed to know exactly the goings-on in every surgical team in his department and every misstep even a medical student might have made.

Even though Dr. Cameron was nearing retirement during my medical school years, he still put in incredible hours. When changing from my scrubs back into my street clothes at the late end of a long OR day, the reasonable chance of running into him prompted me to re-tie my necktie for the walk to my car, even if half the hallways were dark.

His rigor and intensity sparked the same in most around him, I think. He never seemed to be off-guard. I recall running into him once at a movie theater on the weekend. He was on a date with his wife. His white coat had been traded for a suit coat, but he had the same tightly knotted thin tie and starched collar.

Not only did he work long hours on weekdays, but he met every Sunday morning with all the general surgery junior residents. As medical students, we were not invited to these meetings, but we heard about them from the interns with whom we often worked closely. The interns didn't complain about these "Sunday school" sessions. I was never sure if that was because of their confidence that any complaint would somehow become known to the omniscient Dr. Cameron or because they were becoming fully converted to the religion he taught there.

Control, above all self-control, was given the highest premium.

Control required precision, and precision, knowledge.

During the department's morbidity and mortality conferences, held monthly to review surgical complications, I recall other faculty members defending decisions they had made on surgeries. They reported every detail of every lab value and every decisive step in the case in a way that suggested that they also believed in this religion of precision.

Dr. Cameron also met weekly with the rotating medical students. We always sat around a large table in a small room on an upper floor of the hospital. During the rotation, every student was expected to present a short report on a general surgery topic. After each report, Dr. Cameron would comment and expand to a full-table discussion of the topic. Usually, this expanded discussion was in the Socratic method. He would ask questions to individuals, who would either answer correctly or receive a disapproving stare. As no student spoke unless spoken to, one without the correct answer might wait what seemed like minutes before Dr. Cameron would disappointedly redirect his question to someone else.

It wasn't an altogether frightening experience, as he was generally warm and encouraging to students; it was just intense. My clearest recollection from those meetings was one departure from the silent waiting that usually followed his questions. One of my classmates had finished a five-minute presentation on the diagnosis and management of acute appendicitis, another diagnosis that cannot wait for gold standard confirmation.

"Eighty-five percent!" Dr. Cameron stridently declared, before my classmate even inhaled to begin to answer a question about the specificity of a CT scan for diagnosing acute appendicitis.

"And what is the specificity of clinical examination *alone* to diagnose acute appendicitis?" he next asked, before immediately answering again. "Eighty-five percent!"

"If you are a general surgeon," he continued, "your pathologist better find a normal appendix in every six you remove for suspected appendicitis. If not, then you are missing some." Dr.

Cameron went on to suggest that a surgeon ordering a CT scan to make a diagnosis that she should make with her hands should rethink her career choice.[5]

At that moment, I finally understood the tie, the short hair, the almost overly rigorous hours. Some weighty matters, like one-out-of-six appendectomies performed for an incorrect diagnosis, were totally outside of Dr. Cameron's control. That fact only redoubled his efforts to control what he could control.

Dr. Cameron managed uncertainty in diagnosis, especially in the time-pressured setting of possible acute appendicitis, by emphasizing his own personal accountability. In the moment, with the patient's bared belly palpated by his own fingers, he would *decide* the diagnosis. He would divide the gray into black and white because he had to. Nobody else --- least of all some expensive CT scanner --- was going to do it for him.

Imperious

As much as I admire Dr. Cameron's sense of accountability, not everyone agrees that his method is the best way to diagnose acute appendicitis. I have also seen a physician's overemphasis of personal responsibility create as many challenges as it fixed.

An intern on the general surgery team at the time, I called my professor on a Saturday morning to report that a consult team had recommended an invasive test on one of her surgical patients, a Mr. Bledsoe, who was having some mild breathing problems.

"You stopped it, right?" she replied.

"It wasn't to happen during the weekend anyway," I explained. "They scheduled it for Monday morning."

"But you stopped it ... right?"

Through the phone, I could feel Dr. MacArthur's wrath building until she could hold it in no longer.

"Listen, are you helping me or hurting me? It is enough for me to deal with incompetent consulting teams. I don't need *you* trying to hurt my patients as well."

Forcing calm to my voice, I responded, "I told them that I

would check with you to be sure, but that they should not order it because I expected that you wouldn't want it done."

"Not want it! Are you kidding? Why would anyone be so foolish as to order a test that has those risks attached? Why am I the only one looking out for my patients? Did they order it or not? Forget what they tell you. Check with nursing. Check with radiology. Make sure that there is no way that Bledsoe goes down to radiology on Monday morning."

"I will," I stated, as I heard the phone click on the other end.

I called radiology scheduling and left messages. I called the radiologist on call and asked her to remove the order from their list. She made a note to pass it on to the team on Monday. I spoke again with the medicine consult team and made it clear that under no circumstances was Mr. Bledsoe to have the test Monday morning.

Mr. Bledsoe's nurse and I reviewed the plan again Monday morning during rounds.

"Just make sure that he doesn't leave the unit for any reason," I said. "I have a bad feeling about this one. Evil forces seem to conspire against MacArthur's patients."

The nurse chuckled, knowingly.

I didn't.

Even the unit clerk sitting at the front desk was aware that Mr. Bledsoe shouldn't be checked out to a patient transporter headed to radiology for this cancelled test.

I was operating with Dr. MacArthur that day. Her OR was intense enough without the additional stress of the weekend's fiasco hanging over her.

You must understand that Dr. MacArthur wasn't a bad physician. Her heart was in the right place, I think. Most had a hard time seeing her heart, but I do think she had good intentions. She just practiced in a different way. She lived the adage frequently touted in general surgery that "only the paranoid survive," but she took that paranoia to another level than most. Her baseline assumption was that everyone involved in the care of her patients was trying to hurt them. Only *she* stood between her patients and disaster at every moment. Rather than seeking and welcoming consensus, she alone knew.

My pager, lying on the desk in the corner, went off during our second surgery. The nurse didn't disturb Dr. MacArthur to ask if I wanted the page answered. No one disturbs Dr. MacArthur during surgery if one can avoid it.

When we finished the case, Dr. MacArthur went over to the desk to complete her paperwork for the case. The sound that escaped her somehow comingled an explosion, a fervent declaration of complete exasperation, and the violent death of an animal, all in one. From my position, helping the anaesthesiologist wheel the surgical patient's bed through the door, I saw Dr. MacArthur pull a piece of scratch paper out from the belt clip of my pager, which still lay on the desk.

Everyone in the room froze.

By the time I had taken a couple of steps closer to the desk, I saw the note that she held up for me.

"Radiology report: Bledsoe study --- negative."

I need not describe the events of the next few minutes.

Two hours later, after finishing our third surgery for the day, I was able to slip over to the unit where our patients' rooms were. Dr. MacArthur had already blown through. Everyone looked shell-shocked.

From Mr. Bledsoe's nurse and the clerk, I heard sincere apologies. They knew I would bear the brunt of MacArthur's wrath. I also heard explanations. The nurse offered, "At the shift change, I heard that this test was cancelled from the outgoing nurse, but when they came for him, they said that MacArthur had ordered a test. There is no way that I was going to call Dr. MacArthur or do anything other than speed her patient along."

The clerk similarly had heard the warning at shift change, but when the orderly signed the patient out for transport, he wasn't about to question anything on a MacArthur patient.

I called the radiologist who performed the study.

"How did you perform a test without a requisition?" I asked. "How many times have you guys postponed studies I *wanted* because no one could find our requisition form?"

"There wasn't any requisition, which I thought was strange, but I just did you a favor and filled it out myself."

"Why didn't you page me?"

"We all know MacArthur. No way am I going to call her OR and ask about anything."

Even the radiology scheduler broke protocol. He reviewed the weekend's messages in reverse order, hearing my cancellation of the study before hearing of the request for it from the internal medicine consult team. Only the latter mentioned Dr. MacArthur's name specifically. He knew better than to raise questions about her patients, even having never met her.

Thankfully, Mr. Bledsoe fared well. He experienced no complications from the test itself. The negative test result proved even more definitively that he didn't need it, but at least no harm was done.

Only this perfect storm of at least four people breaking protocol to avoid alerting Dr. MacArthur could have possibly allowed a multiply cancelled test to happen anyway. I may be wrong, but I felt that Dr. MacArthur's opinion that she alone protected her patients exposed them to much greater danger, even if she fully took responsibility. It functionally fulfilled her suspicion that no one else *was* thinking and doing his best for the patients. She scared all thinking out of the other team members.

Civics and Specifics

An alternative to Dr. Cameron's stringent personal accountability and MacArthur's tyranny is to use a consensus opinion in the process of diagnosis. Drs. Unni and Rosenberg and their expert bone pathologist colleagues may not have agreed with each other well when interpreting those cartilage cases in isolation, but could they have been more consistent if we had them all in the same room? Some critics of that study actually spurned the idea that a pathologist should ever review a cartilaginous lesion case without a surgeon and radiologist present.

These critics argued that the real gold standard for diagnosing cartilaginous lesions is the consensus opinion of what is termed a multi-disciplinary tumor board. They cannot argue that a consensus opinion removes uncertainty in the accuracy of a diagnosis, but it may provide a more consistent diagnosis.

Every week, I meet with just such a tumor board comprised of all the specialists at my cancer center who are involved in the care of sarcoma-type cancers. In these meetings, we review every new suspected sarcoma. Whichever of us met the patient initially in a clinic will present the pertinent details of the patient's story and physical findings. The radiologist will show the imaging studies on a screen and walk through the important findings as well as the range of diagnoses she interprets as consistent with those findings. With or without a drum roll, the pathologist will render his diagnosis by review of the glass slides, including important diagnostic stains, on a microscope that projects its field of view onto a second screen.

Most importantly, at any moment, every person in the room knows that he or she is welcome to ask questions or make suggestions. A surgeon may not have advanced training focused on CT findings, but she certainly brings to the discussion a lot of knowledge of anatomy and experience with looking at CTs of the types of cancers she treats. The medical oncologist has also read the pathology textbooks pertinent to the cancers he treats. The clinic nurse or social worker may have noted a detail from the history that the patient never mentioned when the physician was present. Everyone has something to offer.

Some cases can be reviewed quickly as everyone agrees without hesitation on a diagnosis and treatment plan. At other times, cases are not so clear. A case may be tabled until the next week with a plan to gather more information or receive results from additional tests in the interim.

Like any other diagnostic test, the use of multidisciplinary tumor boards can be and has been tested as to its contribution to accurate diagnosis and more importantly its benefit or risk to patients.[5] As it has been evaluated so far, the practice of having multiple pairs of eyes look at and multiple brains think about cancer cases appears to help improve patient outcomes.

I know that I have changed others' minds and certainly had my own mind changed by such discussions. For complex cancers like so many in the group of entities collectively called sarcoma, such tumor boards may even out the general muddle of uncertainty.

Of course, just as different individual experts may disagree on a diagnosis for a particular case, the consensus among a particular group of practitioners will not necessarily agree with the consensus of another group. Each group's composition matters immensely. The story of the rise and arguable fall of PSA testing illustrates this important point.

When the prostate specific antigen or PSA became a widely available blood test to help assess a man's risk for prostate cancer, urologists began to use it. They measured the strength of the PSA as a test against the gold standard of a pathologist reviewing a prostate biopsy. Luckily, such pathology interpretations are much more consistent for prostate cancer than for cartilaginous lesions.

Clinical scientists pondered the data, crunched the sensitivity and specificity numbers, and picked levels of PSA that posed sufficient risk to recommend biopsy. Just like the bell curves at this chapter's beginning, any threshold they picked would miss some cases and over-diagnose others. Because they always used a second test, in the form of a biopsy, urologists were comfortable with the PSA as a screening test.

A high PSA would prompt biopsy. When biopsy confirmed the presence of prostate cancer, urologists knew how to treat it with aggressive surgery and radiation. They found that PSA screening for prostate cancer was promoting increased length of survival among diagnosed prostate cancer patients. Sounds great, right? Early detection leads to more success with curing the cancer.

The problem was that urologists were treating the prostate cancers diagnosed from biopsies following high PSA levels the same as they had treated the prostate cancers diagnosed from biopsies in the days before PSA screening. As much as the gold standard pathologic diagnosis hadn't specifically changed, its circumstance had changed dramatically. Circumstance or context matters for the pathologic diagnosis of prostate cancer. Context determines what the diagnosis means.

If the circumstance for seeking a pathologic diagnosis of prostate cancer is during autopsies in 80-year-old men who have died of causes unrelated to prostate cancer, the pathologist will diagnose cancer in a majority of the prostates in those otherwise-deceased men.[7] We can all agree that such diagnoses mean very little to those men specifically. What then does the diagnosis of prostate cancer mean to a man who is 80, otherwise healthy, who underwent prostate biopsy because of a high PSA on routine screening? The fact that most men over 80 have prostate cancer and will die of something completely unrelated may mean that we should not get too worked up about that diagnosis. We can't be sure.

Expanding these principles across a population, some began to ask an important question. Are we actually diagnosing prostate cancer at an earlier, more treatable stage, or just an earlier stage? Are we perhaps just diagnosing a disease with a long and slow natural course at early stages of that course? If the pathologic diagnosis of prostate cancer prior to PSA screening meant that the man had a deadly disease with a fifty-fifty chance of surviving five years, does catching it earlier by two years and rendering a fifty-fifty chance of survival at seven years accomplish anything? One might even criticize that it gives the man diagnosed two extra years of the anxiety of impending death. They call this particular phenomenon lead-time bias. In other words, we are skewing our perceived survival from time of diagnosis by earlier detection. We are not actually detecting disease at a time when its natural course can be changed by intervention.

What should we do with this information? Well, the consensus opinion will depend entirely upon who contributes to the consensus. PSA screening sparks fierce debate among physicians. This isn't new. I recall more than one professor of mine in medical school, more than a decade ago, declaring that he would never allow his PSA to be tested. Other professors taught us that we should test PSA levels on every man over fifty if we intended to be good physicians.

The professors who taught us the value of PSA testing were urologists, the surgeons whose practices are filled by men with high PSA levels needing biopsy and treatment. The professors who denigrated the PSA practiced in other fields. I am not suggesting that the urologists who believed in PSA screening were only interested in their business; they also had likely had more personal and more painful experiences with prostate cancer diagnosed too late to be helped. The point is that even a consensus opinion will depend on its contributors. In recent news, many physicians have begun publicly to denounce the PSA as a screening test. The Urological Association of America disagrees.

The Anatomy of Gray

Every diagnostic test has flaws. Physicians test tests to characterize these flaws, hoping to render test results as known unknowns, rather than unknown unknowns. We compare tests to gold standards, even if those standards evolve over time. When we lack gold standards, we compare expert opinions to each other to learn how consistent they can be. Time will teach the ultimate value of the tests we employ at the beginning of a disease course. We watch the passage of time with some trepidation because some diagnoses become less treatable as they become more certain.

Some physicians manage the uncertainty of diagnosis by emphasizing personal responsibility. Others invoke a consensus of experts or a multidisciplinary care team. The membership of that team will impact its consensus opinion. The next chapter will discuss the contributions and interactions of the two most important members of that team, the patient and the treating physician. In this chapter's last story I will give you an example of a particularly difficult diagnosis toward which my patient and I struggled together, having no absolute results from which to work.

Brandy was a patient referred for evaluation of a painful lesion in the bone at the base of her right big toe. Cross-country running through the mountains was her pastime, hobby, and first pursuit after her work. She had run a 5K high-altitude race the week before, but noted severe toe pain on the final 100 yards of the race. The pain persisted after the race. She called her primary care physician to get a referral to a sports medicine specialist. Radiographs obtained in the sports clinic showed nothing strictly sports-related, but a bone-destroying tumor right at the joint connecting the toe to the foot. The supporting bone of the joint had fractured on the side with the tumor, offering an explanation for the sudden onset of pain during her last race.

Other than the break itself, the lesion in the bone had mixed features, some suggesting more aggressive behavior, and others less aggressive behavior. The tumor had eaten its way completely out of the bone to one side, but only up to the cartilage of the joint, not through it. The first feature suggested a cancer, the second a benign tumor called giant cell tumor of bone.

An MRI obtained before Brandy's coming to my clinic confirmed in three dimensions the features suggested by the two-dimensional radiographs. The MRI also identified a very small, distinct mass under the middle of the foot, a couple of inches away. This second mass, only about 5 mm in its greatest dimension, had the appearance of another benign condition called fibromatosis. Fibromatosis isn't really a tumor as much as it is a thickening of the muscle-lining tissue layer. Brandy and I decided that since the small second mass was deep and likely unrelated, we would simply remember to check it again with imaging later.

For the toe mass, Brandy came to the operating room. She slept while I made an incision, cut a sample from the bone tumor, packed the wound with gauze temporarily and brought the specimen to the pathology room. The technician there froze the sample. He then placed some shavings from it on glass slides and stained them.

"So clinically, this looks like a giant cell tumor?" the pathologist asked, while turning on her microscope and placing the still-wet glass slides onto its platform.

"Yes and no," I answered. "The overall appearance is most like giant cell tumor of bone, as it has respected the joint itself, but it isn't classic. It destroyed the side of the bone in one direction."

I pulled up the radiographs and MRI on the nearby computer for her to see, while she perused the slide.

"It all looks pretty bland," she said, frowning into the microscope eyepieces. "I just don't see many giant cells."

I peered into the other pair of eye-pieces on the other side of the desk and agreed, "Nothing high-grade, certainly."

"No, there is really nothing that looks at all scary in this, there are just no. . . . Well, there's one giant cell there. Yes, just not many giant cells. Maybe it is burned out?"

By this she referred to the state in which some tumors have

spontaneously and inexplicably fizzled-out, stopped growing, and been replaced by scar-like tissue.

"Well, the only way she noticed it was sudden toe pain, which I am guessing started from that fracture there." I pointed to radiographs on the screen. "That happened during a 5K she was running a week and a half ago. I guess it could have been there a long time, burned out, and then became newly aggravated with the fracture. Still, that doesn't explain the soft-tissue extension, which looks a bit more aggressive."

"Is maybe *part* of it more aggressive? What part do we have on this slide? From where in the tumor did your sample come?"

"The thing is so small; I would be surprised if it had different parts. Anyway, the part we sampled for pathology and are looking at here includes the most aggressive part on the imaging, as that was what we came to first."

"I really think this is a nothing. Due to the overall picture, I favor giant cell. There is certainly no malignancy, whatever it is. Let me see who else is up in the offices to see if other opinions can shed some light on this."

She took the slide from the microscope platform, and we rode a nearby elevator up to the faculty offices for the pathology department.

Once on the upper floor, we walked the slides into the office at the end of the hall. Usually, our sarcoma pathologist is one of the first to arrive in the morning, so we expected him to be there. He didn't disappoint us.

"Yes, I agree. Nothing on here looks high-grade malignant," the sarcoma pathologist noted while viewing the slides through his scope. "There aren't many giant cells, but there don't have to be a lot of giant cells to call it giant cell tumor of bone. This might have just burned out and would have gone away entirely if she hadn't fractured it. Can you get us more tissue before you close? The final diagnosis may be tough."

"Sure, I can do that," I said. "Because of the location, even if this is something worse than giant cell tumor of bone, nothing I do today will open or remove the possibility of salvaging that toe. From the fracture alone, whatever this is, it is already in the joint and therefore surrounding the base of the toe. I'll just remove all of it for you."

While scribbling some notes on the slip of paper that accompanied the slides, the pathologist concluded, "Then I will sign this out: no evidence of malignancy; favor giant cell tumor of bone; defer to permanent."

"Done. Thanks."

I left the office and took the elevator back down to the OR level, where Brandy awaited me, patiently asleep. I scrubbed my hands again and donned a fresh gown and gloves.

"What was it?" the scrub tech asked. "Is it bad?"

"Hard to say. It doesn't look scary at all. All the cells were bland. I only worry about their shape."

"What do you mean?"

The surgical fellow joined the conversation while we extended our incision a few millimeters in each direction and began scooping the rest of the small mass out of the bone cavity it had created in the toe.

"Well, I can show you the slides afterwards. The cells were just a little round for my liking."

"So?"

"So, what kind of cells should comprise the background cells of a giant cell tumor?"

"They should be spindle cells with the nuclei matching the nuclei of the giant cells." He rattled the correct answer off easily.

"Well, the cells were not spindle cells. They were not scary, but they were not spindled either."

"So?"

"So, the only cancers I know of that are aggressively malignant without having ugly-looking other features are epithelioid sarcomas."

"Aren't they supposed to start in the soft tissues?" the fellow asked.

"Yes."

"But?"

He could tell that his pat answer didn't dismiss my concern.

"But this lesion doesn't classically fit any diagnosis. I hope it is just a burned-out giant cell tumor, as the pathologists favor for today. I am just not yet convinced. There are too many funny things about it. It's my job --- and soon to be yours, about 8 months from now --- to worry about the worst-case scenario. From the information we have right now, some odd variant of an epithelioid sarcoma best fits that worst-case-scenario."

We finished scraping and used a burr to deepen the cavity in the bone in all directions, a technique intended to remove the final vestiges of benign tumors such as giant cell tumor.

"Look at the way it respected the articular cartilage," I noted.

The cartilage was a mere wafer of rubbery white dividing the cavity where the tumor had been to one side from the joint space on the other. All the bone up to it on the defect side had been completely destroyed, but the cartilage was left perfectly intact.

"Well, that fits with giant cell, burnt out or not," I said. "This, on the other hand, does not." I indicated the erosion through the cortical bone to one side. "I don't like that. You add a little too aggressive behavior to a little too bland histology, and my head scratching leads me to think about things that can be aggressive without looking aggressive under a microscope. I know it's crazy; it's just my paranoid-for-this-patient hunch. We'll see what the final path shows next week."

We filled the defect with small granules of bone graft and sutured the wounds closed.

We didn't get the final pathology result until the following week, as it required a couple of consultations from outside pathologists.

Our pathologist called me to summarize: "It has epithelioid features and too many mitotic figures, but there has never been a epithelioid sarcoma reported to start in the bone. And even if that were a recognized diagnosis, this doesn't fit perfectly."

Of the two consulting pathologists, one called it epithelioid sarcoma and recommended foot amputation, but gave little argument for this essentially creative diagnosis. The second hedged more, agreeing with descriptively epithelioid features, but not willing to argue that it should be treated so drastically.

Brandy came to my office to discuss her options.

"As you know, there are details of this diagnosis that remain seriously in question but will likely remain in question permanently," I began. "That gives you and me three options. We can simply watch this closely. We can remove the toe up high near the middle of the foot. Or we can remove your foot."

"I have to admit that if I do anything other than watch it, I'm inclined to choose the amputation," she answered. "I've been reading about it since our last conversation, and I think you're right. There are many people who seem to argue that missing my big toe that high might be worse for athletics than having my whole foot off. No matter what, I need a little time to think. Is waiting another couple of weeks very dangerous?"

"No. I don't think so. By two weeks from today, it will have been four weeks from the date of your first foot MRI. Let's plan on your coming to see me that day after a new MRI of the entire limb and chest CT that morning. It may give us more information about the other small soft-tissue mass that we initially thought was low risk. We can also rule out any other masses in the limb, given the regional spread that can characterize epithelioid sarcoma."

Brandy returned to the clinic with a completely healed toe wound and feeling very little pain. No disease had been noted elsewhere up the leg or in the lungs. The MRI, however, showed that the tiny, suspected fibromatosis had quadrupled in size over four weeks. It was still small and still causing no symptoms, but markedly larger.

"I don't think we can ignore this other lesion anymore," I cautioned. "I hate to keep giving you anaesthetics, but the radiologist won't be able to needle-biopsy something that small."

"Well, I still haven't completely decided what I want to do anyway. Let's do a biopsy of the little lump. Then I'll have all possible information."

Two days later found Brandy again patiently asleep on the operating table while I took another set of slides up the elevator to the top floor.

"I still can't say for sure what name belongs on this, but it looks exactly like the tissue you scraped out of that toe," the pathologist concluded.

After final slides and all of the special stains were available for this second mass, his opinion hadn't changed.

When Brandy returned to my office, she read the frustration

in my face.

"So nothing changed from the frozen section?"

"No," I answered. "This looks like the same epithelioid-like tissue."

"But now it is in two places in my foot, one of them having grown rapidly over only a month."

"Yes." I agreed. "I don't think that we will have the privilege of any black-and-white answers in your case, but that makes multiple gray arrows pointing toward something dangerous."

"I have been reading about epithelioid sarcomas," she said. "This is how they spread."

"Yes. This is what concerns me, too."

"I am ready to have my foot off before we find this any further up," Brandy concluded.

"It's the decision I would make for myself. As much as I don't want this to be a real cancer for you, finding the same thing growing in two places makes the decision a bit easier, truth be told."

We didn't know with certainty that these two tumors in Brandy's foot represented cancer. We will never know, unless the outcome I most hope not to see --- disease relapse in the lungs or further up the leg --- occurs in Brandy's case. We have no gold standard to test her test results against. Brandy and I managed the uncertainty wrought by the absence of a black-and-white answer with a decision to believe the diagnosis to which multiple gray arrows pointed.

Brandy's lesion was a little too aggressive on radiographs and in terms of bone destruction seen during the first surgery to call it benign. The cells had a fried-egg roundness to them that suggested epithelioid to everyone who saw them. If nothing else, this feature points to a dangerous and often deceptively bland-looking lesion; it appeared in two locations in the foot, one that grew rapidly over a very brief time interval. We certainly could have waited for time to make things even clearer, but instead reached a consensus to move forward, well aware that we'd never know the truth with certainty.

Multiple gray arrows pointing in one direction don't make a black-and-white diagnosis, but they can lead us to *choose* a diagnosis and move forward through the fog.

Starting Your Conversation. . . .

Positive Results

Principle: Test results are never perfect. We measure the accuracy of tests against some accepted standard definition of each disease.

Ask your physician: Does this test generally err on the side of over-diagnosis or under-diagnosis?

Standards & Poor

Principle: The gold-standard definitions of disease change over time as technology and knowledge change.

Ask your physician: How has the definition of my condition changed over the years? Were the diagnostic methods used a decade ago identifying the same patients as the methods today?

Competing Catechisms

Principle: The best definition we have for some diseases is no better than an expert opinion. Sometimes even expert opinions don't agree.

Ask your physician: How much experience does the radiologist or pathologist interpreting my case have with the particular diagnosis he is making? Would I get the same diagnosis if my case was reviewed by his equal in another medical center?

Thorned Roses

Principle: We often pick and choose among conflicting results what we will believe, which will prompt action.

Ask your physician: Do any of my test results point away from our working diagnosis? How will our decisions now affect our ability to go back and test another diagnosis later?

Compartmentalizing

Principle: Some diagnoses will never be confirmable, even with time, because intervention removes the opportunity to know the truth.

Ask your physician: Will we become more confident of my diagnosis over time, or is this as confident as we will have opportunity to be?

Keeping the Faith

Principle: Some physicians address uncertainty in diagnosis by emphasizing personal responsibility and rigor.

Ask your physician: If I am determined to do my part to get better as a patient, what will that look like? What can I do to help?

Imperious

Principle: A physician's sense of personal responsibility can impede good care if he fails to encourage contribution from every potential team member.

Ask your physician: Who are the members of the team that will help you take care of me?

Civics and Specifics

Principle: When hard black-and-white answers and test results are impossible, sometimes we turn to multiple opinions to build a consensus instead. Who contributes to that consensus can change it dramatically.

Ask your physician: With whom will you discuss my case?

The Anatomy of Gray

Principle: Sometimes we build a consensus diagnosis from multiple test results rather than multiple opinions.

Ask your physician: What additional tests might increase our confidence that this is the correct way to go?

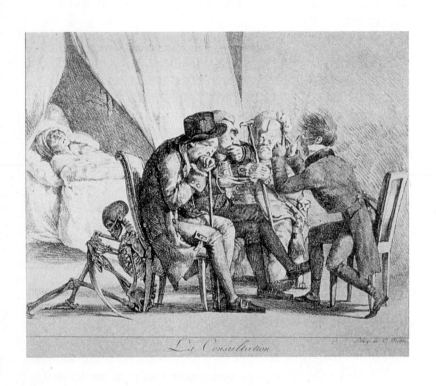

La Consultation

IDENTIFY THE PROBLEM

Watching P's and Q's

"This is a 39-year-old female, bounced back from an admission two weeks ago for critical hypokalemia."

The intern began her formal presentation to the rounding team physicians on the first day of my internal medicine rotation during medical school. She had admitted the patient the night before.

"This time, she was found on the ground by her teenage son who called an ambulance to bring her to the ER. He didn't come along with her, and she hasn't woken up enough yet to permit the taking of a history. She arrived with an electrolyte disturbance similar to last time, which we're correcting."

"She has a history of a terrible eating disorder," another intern said. "I remember her from last time. On her last admission, she confessed that she had taken diuretics for weight loss."

Diuretics are prescription medicines used to treat high blood pressure by causing salt wasting into the urine. Their use by individuals obsessed with weight loss is considered one of the most severe manifestations of eating disorders, like anorexia or bulimia. Someone willing to take --- in illegal fashion --- such potentially dangerous medications for the sole purpose of weight-loss simply cannot be thinking clearly.

"But she never admitted to making herself vomit during her last admission," the intern added. "Even when we had her directly observed, she never was caught trying to gag herself or try anything else funny, prior to a vomiting episode."

This patient's admissions to the hospital the night before and two weeks prior resulted from loss of consciousness due to a severe imbalance of salts in her circulation. She specifically had hypokalemia, or low potassium. It had become clear on her last admission that her low potassium was caused by a couple of weeks of excessive vomiting. She had been suspected on that admission of having bulimia, a severe eating disorder often associated with self-induced vomiting. She had never admitted to it on their repeated questioning.

"Remember, bulimia is ultimately a psychiatric disease. I figured last time that she was so convinced that food was evil, that she didn't even need to gag herself anymore to induce vomiting," the other resident reasoned.

"Since she was neither suicidal nor homicidal, we couldn't admit her to the psychiatric ward without her consent. She refused to give it repeatedly. She wanted to get back to work," concluded the intern.

"So she's back again even worse than last time" a third resident interjected, shaking her head. "She's going to come back in a box next time."

The lead physician on the team turned to me.

"Kevin, why don't you take this patient, for starters? If she wakes up this afternoon as her electrolytes normalize, try to get a history. We need to understand what is keeping her from letting us get her the psychiatric help she needs."

It was actually the following day when Barbara awoke enough to permit conversation. She didn't recall any of the circumstances surrounding her being brought to the hospital. She did talk about the two weeks she had been at home between hospitalizations.

"Those pills they gave me last time, they make me so sick," she began. "I kept trying to take them but couldn't keep them down. I would take them, and then throw up an hour later. Up would come the little red capsules." Barbara was referring to the potassium replacement pills she had been given to take at home. "They told me that tomatoes and orange juice also had potassium, so all I've eaten since going home is V8 and orange juice. I can't keep solids down, so I keep trying the juices. I got a case of each."

"Why do you think that you keep throwing up?" I asked.

"I just feel so sick. And I can't afford to be sick. I'm going to lose my job at the factory if I don't get better and get back to work."

"That sounds like a lot of stress in your life right now. You're worried about a lot of things." I decided to hit the eating problem head-on. "Are you worried about your weight, too?"

"My weight? Yes. I'm worried that I can't eat enough to keep my weight up, since nothing stays down."

"Are you trying to stay thin?"

"No. I don't have time to worry about the way I look. Sure, I worried about that like all girls do back in my early twenties. I tried dieting. It wasn't for me."

"Are you taking medications to help your dieting?"

"Once, years ago, I picked up some of those dietetic pills from the pharmacy."

"Do you mean diuretic pills?"

"Yeah, the type to help reduce your hunger. I forget which brand; it was Trim Fast or something like that."

The longer I spoke with Barbara, the more the image of a self-destructive bulimic in denial of her problem melted away. She might not articulate her story well, but she was, basically, honest. And she didn't have bulimia. Her story ultimately pointed toward other causes for her vomiting, once we believed it. She had heartburn, worsening over the last year, that she attributed to stress related to her husband's leaving and her son's getting more deeply into trouble at school and otherwise. Only for the last month, two weeks prior to her first hospitalization, had she begun to vomit an hour or so after eating. The problem began intermittently at first, but ultimately followed every meal.

On further investigation, we learned that she had what was once a much more common problem, though recently rare. She had developed an ulcer and subsequently a near complete obstruction of the outflow from her stomach into the small intestine. The high potassium diet she had diligently pursued to get better had probably worsened rather than improved her condition. Almost exclusive consumption of orange juice and V8 may deliver some potassium, but their acidity didn't help settle her ulcer down.

We transferred Barbara to the care of a surgical team that corrected the obstruction of her stomach outlet. She started taking appropriate medications to prevent further ulcers and returned to home and work as good as new.

I often reflect on this case. How did Barbara's diagnosis get so blatantly missed on her first admission, two weeks before I met her? How did her history of taking a relatively harmless diet pill get mistaken --- simply by her poor articulation --- for a history of diuretic use and a sign of a very concerning, life-threatening eating disorder?

It wasn't from a lack of skill or knowledge on the part of her physicians. I have never since encountered a more intelligent, dedicated team of physicians as that particular group. As a rule, they were uncommonly thorough, as well as exceptionally knowledgeable. Internal medicine residents at Johns Hopkins Hospital have nicknamed themselves the "Osler Marines," testament to the rigor and intensity of those who pursue training in the program begun by the famous physician Sir William Osler. How was this particular battalion of Osler Marines so profoundly mistaken on its first interaction with Barbara?

I think it comes down to trust.

As soon as we learned to trust and rethink her story on that second admission, the diagnosis followed and guided successful therapy.

The question then becomes, why didn't they trust her the first time?

I could surmise that it was because Barbara was working class, rough around the edges, lacking developed articulation of her story. To counter this explanation, the vast majority of the patients those residents interview, examine, and treat, have no more education than Barbara.

Many have much less.

It might also be said that the number of desperate and self-dangerous heroin addicts treated by the Osler medicine service might lead its "Marines" to expect to mistrust patients. They still rarely failed to get the critical points of a patient's history correct. There was more to this story.

Although the many drug addicts admitted to the hospital for their variety of infections and other problems quite definitively engage in self-destructive behaviors, most don't *intend* to harm themselves. Eating disorders are different. The team first met Barbara when she was nearly comatose in an ER, suffering from vomiting-induced electrolyte disturbances so severe that survivability was in question. One small mistaken detail like "diuretic" rather than "dietetic" pill for weight-loss raised suspicions that were very difficult to subdue. The mere conception of a potential diagnosis such as an eating disorder can be a complete game-changer to the diagnostic process. It introduces an element of inherent mistrust of the patient.

I think in Barbara's case, all of these factors swirled and conspired against her: her poor situation, the ingrained sense of guarded trust with which Osler medicine residents must approach all their patients, the potential diagnosis of a condition which includes dishonesty to self and self-destructive thoughts and behaviors. Ultimately, it took a medical student with far less knowledge, less experience with manipulative patients, and far more time available to sit and listen to the patient for the rest of the story to come to light.

The diagnostic process critically depends on clear communication between physicians and patients. Everyone talks about bedside manner. Many use this to refer to the kindness or compassion shown by a physician. I am not confident that a physician's kindness or compassion matters all that much. What matters more is communication. A physician must receive communication from and offer clear communication to his patients. Failing to communicate effectively creates even more uncertainty than that of any other diagnostic test.

Losing the Game

As I sat in the workroom of my clinic and reviewed the documents from her prior physician, I looked forward to meeting Anna less and less. As cut-and-dried and sometimes boring as most medical charts and notes are to review, there can be a tone apparent. I liked neither the tone I read in Anna's physician's note, nor what it implied about her. The tone comes some from the words chosen to express the information, but more from the patterns of information recorded.

Many in the medical world joke that medical student histories include everything from recent travelogues of patients' vacations to the bowel habits of their household pets. Notes recorded by anyone more senior than a third-year medical student will display the writer's thinking in the facts recorded. Physicians document what are called pertinent positive and pertinent negative details, not everything and the kitchen sink. A medical note isn't a court of law, where all sides of an argument are given equal sway. More like a crafted law brief, the recorded details usually build toward an argument. One can guess the punch line long before the note specifically states it in the Impression or Assessment section at the end.

The selection of facts to record or leave out requires judgment. Excellent physicians judge what importantly informs the identification of a patient's problem, and what is extraneous, superfluous information. Physicians don't always reserve their judgment for the diagnosis alone; they also judge and build arguments to support their judgments of patient personalities. As I reviewed Anna's medical record, I received the distinct impression building of a patient not to be trusted, a patient using the system with ulterior motives.

Some patients use the uncertainties in healthcare to accomplish their own agendas. Medical issues bear such sway legally that great authority is afforded a final medical diagnosis and plan. This circumstance in and of itself isn't a problem; but as they say, power corrupts, and absolute power corrupts absolutely.

Every human culture of which I am aware grants incredible leeway to the ill. Legally, our nation's economy spends over 50 billion dollars each year to support a system to compensate workers injured on the job.[1] Our Federal government financially supports with life-long social security checks anyone whom it has medically deemed to be permanently disabled.

Aside from these bureaucracies and legalities, we all offer the ill a large dose of understanding. We are never as demanding of sick family members. We pamper them to the best of our capacities. I don't criticize the fact that individuals temporarily or permanently disabled by illness are given special treatment. That is as it should be. The problem arises when individuals seek these special treatments in the absence of actual disablement. Secondary gain, or the benefit associated with a sick role, is discussed at great length in the psychology of disease.

Some have mastered the skill --- either to their own benefit or detriment, depending on your perspective --- of establishing themselves in this sick role without actually being disabled. Most are not evil, lying thieves. Most are people unhappy with some other aspect of their lives that remains unaddressed. They may have a terribly disappointing or abusive home, work, or social environment that they escape through the sick role.

Whatever their subconscious reason, they tend toward the most uncertain areas of medicine. They find in themselves the diagnoses that are most difficult to refute with hard diagnostic facts.

In orthopaedics, these patients populate back pain and shoulder pain clinics. More generally, they gravitate toward the odd and controversial diagnoses such as chronic fatigue syndrome, reflex sympathetic dystrophy, porphyria, exertional compartment syndrome, and fibromyalgia. Not to say that everyone diagnosed with these conditions is gaming the system. Far from it, but these diagnoses on some level are difficult to rule out conclusively. One part of medicine rife with these agenda-driven patients is the care of patients injured while at work.

Many injuries happen on the job. Most injured workers receive treatment in uneventful fashion and return to the workforce. In some cases, patients disagree with employers on the details regarding if and when they should return to work and how disabled their injuries have left them. While some of these sticky situations derive from bad employers, others arise from bad workers. Physicians can feel uncomfortable in either case, as they are often caught in the middle, mistrusted by both parties. They also know that their medical record and decision-making will almost certainly become a document with legal implications. Judges and courts and perhaps even juries will review their documentation.

When an injury has happened at work without prompting legal battles, the treating physician will invariably include the location-of-injury detail in the history recorded. In contrast, legal wrangling over disputed disability arising from an injury of any type sustained while at work dramatically alters the documentation. Rather than noting once somewhere in the first history that the injury occurred in the work place, every following note will also include this notation early, if not in the very first line. "This patient is a #-year-old woman who was injured at work," opens each document. One often even loses a sense for what actual diagnosis resulted from the injury. The patient becomes *diagnosed* with a "work injury, not otherwise specified." The follow-up notes will more likely detail the date and circumstance of the accident, rather than the injury that resulted.

With this, we return to Anna's medical record.

Anna was a "26-year-old female injured at work on June 31st, 2009 when she lifted a bar of steel." Only much later did the note mention that her ongoing complaint had been low back pain, rather than, say, a broken leg or arm. She had become one of those diagnosed (legally, more than medically) with an injury at work. Her referring physician's note expressed frustration with Anna's persistent lack of improvement over months of physical therapy. Anna required narcotic prescriptions for longer than he either expected or approved. He clearly doubted that her "work injury" was to blame for her pain. His later notes began to mention chronic back pain. These later notes communicated that he thought the pain had preceded her injury. The tone of a frustrated physician who didn't trust his patient was clear.

To compound the tone of frustration, Anna's physician had noted allergies to a few pain drugs. Such drug allergies can flag that someone has been gaming the system. True allergic reactions to medications are rare. Most true allergic reactions arise to antibiotics or other very large, biologically derived molecules. True allergies to narcotic analgesics are extremely rare. Even when these notations communicate legitimately adverse reactions to a drug or drugs, most are not actually allergies. Some patients, trying to game the system, know that if they claim allergies to certain lighter-duty narcotic pain medications, they can convince physicians to prescribe stronger versions.

While I could not yet be certain that my interaction with Anna would be difficult, the documents convinced me that her referring physician didn't enjoy his. Was he just dumping this patient on me to deal with her chronic back pain?

"Well, I have an easy fix for that," I thought to myself. "A couple of imaging tests to confirm the absence of anything scary, and Anna will be out of my world and back into his."

After reviewing all the notes quickly, I slipped the CD with her imaging into the computer. Imaging could not expose the same tone, could it? The list of studies on the CD flashed on the screen after a few clicks. Imaging might not have a tone in the images, but the pattern of its ordering can. This CD contained only one image, and that from an anteroposterior radiograph (front to back x-ray image) of the lumbar spine. The odd thing was the date on this first and only radiograph; it was less than a week old.

I flipped back through the notes again to see if I had missed some other imaging reports. Sometimes referring physician offices will only send the actual images of the most recent study, but will usually send the radiology reports from all of them. I hadn't missed any. The records included 10 clinic notes, spanning eight months since the first note, the day after the lifting incident at work. There were two pages of laboratory tests, both from that first visit, showing normal blood counts and urinalysis. At the very bottom of the clipped packet, the last page displayed the radiology report for the lone radiograph of the lumbar spine.

The lack of prior imaging surprised me. Of course, most cases of back pain don't require imaging. Most prove to be self-limited episodes that resolve without any significant intervention within 2 to 3 weeks. Pain that lasts longer, most agree, should prompt at least some basic screening imaging in the form of plain radiographs. Usually, referring physicians have erred on the side of ordering too many imaging studies prior to referral to a specialist. With this trend in mind, Anna's referring physician showed admirable restraint. He had avoided an MRI and other expensive imaging on that first visit the day after her injury.

But nothing for eight months?

He hadn't done *nothing*. He had given Anna a few prescriptions of strong narcotic pain pills. He prescribed three different rounds of physical therapy. None of these had helped Anna, according to the notes. The lack of improvement annoyed the physician. Worse than no improvement, her complaints escalated, which frustrated him further. When she complained of sleep disturbance from worsening pain at night, he could no longer dismiss it. On the last visit he had relented and ordered a radiograph.

When the image loaded onto my screen, I felt as if the wheeled desk chair on which I sat had rolled out from underneath me. The radiograph showed an aggressive tumor, eating a hole in the bone of her pelvis and the base of her spine. Not only was Anna a narcotic-seeking, chronic low back pain patient, she also had a very dangerous form of cancer.

How in the world would this workman's comp malingerer cope with the treatment course that she now faced?

A third of the way through nine months of chemotherapy, treatment would stop so Anna could undergo a massive and debilitating surgery to remove half her pelvis and most of the nerve roots from the spine to the lower limb on that side. Tolerating, even surviving, such brutal treatment requires fortuitousness and determination --- I doubted anyone with Anna's history was equal to that.

Although almost angry at the referring physician's likely multi-month delay of diagnosis and treatment initiation, I accepted as mere fact his obvious judgment that Anna was a drug-seeking, system-gaming, agenda-driven patient. This was going to be horrible. In self-pity, I braced myself, cleaned my hands with the requisite sanitizing goop dispensed by each clinic room door, knocked, and entered.

Anna sat quietly in her hospital gown between a woman I guessed to be her mother and a man I guessed to be her boyfriend. The room stank of stale cigarettes from the clothing of one or all three of them.

After introductions --- I was right about the mother, but the boyfriend was actually Anna's husband --- the mother started the conversation.

"Dr. Jones, can you tell us why we were sent here? We got a call telling us to show up at 1:00 PM, but we were a little shocked to find ourselves going to a cancer hospital for an appointment about Anna's back problem. Are you a spine doctor?"

"Do I have cancer?" Anna asked. "I have been telling Dr. Smith for months that I wanted an MRI. He just kept giving me more pain pills and sending me to more PT. I stopped taking them pills months ago. I would flush them as soon as I got 'em home. When I tried taking 'em early on, they made me feel goofy and stopped me up. I would tell him that they made me sick, but he would just give me another kind. I hate 'em all. None of 'em made any difference for the pain. Neither did the PT. Shoot, I could teach you them core-strengthening exercises. They never helped me start sleeping at night or helped me feel better one bit." She paused. "Has it been cancer this whole time? Did lifting that steel bar give me cancer? That wouldn't make sense."

Anna may have been a lot of things that a physician wouldn't like. She smoked. She hadn't finished her high school education. She had a history of bad choices such as illicit-drug experimentation as a teenager. But she wasn't gaming the system in any way. She didn't seek, and in fact discarded (although she worried that she was doing it against medical advice) the prescribed rounds of narcotic analgesics. Far from gaming the system, the system had gamed her, or at least nearly failed her.

By grace alone, her diagnosis happened to be one I could make from relatively objective images and a biopsy that followed. Had the diagnosis depended more heavily on our communication, as most do, my initial bias derived from her prior physician's notes might have prevented my helping her as well.

In the end, Anna tolerated the throes of chemotherapy quite well. It gave her focus enough to quit smoking and improve what she later told me had been a rocky relationship with her husband. She recovered from her --- dare I admit it? --- horrific surgery. She walks very well with her walker, acceptably well with a cane, and even free-handed for short distances. She has never even mentioned suing her prior doctor or her employer over the lifting incident. She is a gracious, appreciative patient.

Once again, poor communication introduced powerful and nearly dangerous uncertainty into the process of diagnosis. The Osler Marines missed Barbara's diagnosis because they thought she was trying to hurt herself. Dr. Smith initially missed Anna's diagnosis because he thought she was trying to help herself to privileges she didn't deserve.

In both cases, the physicians had to begin to doubt themselves before they could trust the patient enough to move toward a diagnosis.

Incongruity

So how did Dr. Smith (and I, initially) misunderstand Anna so egregiously prior to the radiograph? Maybe he is a lousy physician. I doubt it.

Again, it comes down to trust and communication.

He met Anna for evaluation of back pain from an injury sustained at work. Clearly, the injury hadn't been too severe, as it had prompted a clinic visit the next day, not an immediate ambulance trip to an ER. And it was low back pain. According to his later notes and Anna's personal story given to me, the pain was present at some level for weeks before the lifting incident. That means it was already a chronic low back pain, and work comp chronic low back pain at that.

While I don't often see low back pain or workers' compensation patients of any kind in my particular niche practice of sarcoma surgery, I remember the spine clinics from my training in general orthopaedics. I hated them. I literally hated spine clinic.

The teaching physicians with whom I worked were great. The nurses who staffed the spine clinics were patient, kind and skilled, superb in every way. I even enjoyed the technical aspects of the surgeries that were indicated from some patients in those clinics. I enjoyed the satisfying successes we saw in some follow-up patients returning for regular checks.

What I hated were interactions with chronic low back pain patients.

I hated clinic interactions with these patients as a group because I generally like patients, trust patients, and want to help patients find answers to their concerns. Too many (definitely not all) in this group waited in the clinic room with an agenda.

I hated the fact that I entered every new encounter in that clinic with my guard and skepticism on highest alert. To some extent, I had to ignore what they said, instead focusing on what I could find in the clinical examination and imaging. The patient's story and symptoms matter in spine evaluations, but I could not fully trust them. I hated that daunting necessity of mistrust.

I am not alone in mistrusting these encounters. There is even a science that goes into the uncovering of agenda-driven patients. Dr. Gordon Waddell developed and published in 1980 what he called the signs of incongruity.[2] He felt these signs represented evidence for a psychological component to a patient's chronic back pain. These include pain inconsistent and out of proportion with the physical examination; pain to light touch; tenderness, sensory changes, or muscle weakness crossing regions unrelated by the anatomy of nerves; pain on an obvious straight-leg raise that isn't reproduced when the patient is sitting and distracted; pain on simulated rotation that keeps the shoulders and hips (and therefore spine) moving as one unit; pain elicited by pressing down on the patient's head.

One of the teaching physicians with whom I worked in the spine clinic had his own somewhat humorous additions to these, such as the wearing of dark sunglasses in the clinic room, using a hand-carved cane for mobilization, and personalization of the pain: "She gets me right there!" He had grown almost callous to these agenda-ed patients. He quickly saw through and even chuckled at their varied schemes. I could laugh a little with him, but I hated that my interviews with patients in that clinic were more a game of cat and mouse than an honest conversation.

Maybe this was the beginning of Anna's physician's error. He had decided early on that this would be an adversarial relationship. Anna hadn't helped by being less than upfront about her discarding of the pain medicines. Would he have believed her if she had mentioned it?

Maybe he would have had she asked directly for no more.

Although I didn't dwell on this thought with her, the tumor likely would have been discovered months earlier had he ordered the MRI Anna thought she was requesting. Why didn't he order it?

Well, there's the rub.

I have previously discussed some of the many possible findings of uncertain significance on a spine MRI. To the ordering physician personally, diagnostic tests with non-specific --- call them "extra" --- results present no problems. Problems arise while explaining those nonspecific results to a patient, especially to a patient either feeling woefully disenfranchised or actually intent upon gaming the system.

Someone desperately searching for something concrete for the attorney to show a jury will not delight in a negative result, as someone wanting not to have a serious diagnosis will. These diagnosis-hungry patients delight even less in results that sound meaningful on the diagnostic report but are explained to be nothing by the ordering physicians. As necessary as they may be, these explanations raise suspicions and mistrust on the patients' part and devour much of the physician's precious time.

It takes a long time to explain to a patient that the entire focus of the radiology report on an otherwise normal MRI is describing in detail an entity that the physician believes has no bearing on the debilitating pain. Some patients, agenda-ed or not, are so desperate for an answer that they will latch on to such a finding as *the* reason for all their discomfort and unhappiness. Telling that patient that the only objective finding identified in their determined drive for a diagnosis is a finding with no objective interpretation can crush them.

Maybe Dr. Smith was short on time. Maybe he didn't want to disappoint Anna. I can analyze it up and down, but no matter when the specific flaw took root in his thinking, or from what reasoning it sprang, essentially, he passed judgment too quickly. This quick judgment on the patient only extended the uncertainty in her diagnosis.

The Last Shall Be First

As I mentioned, any physician more experienced than a third-year medical student won't record every possible detail of history from the patient that can be gleaned in 90 minutes of questioning. While selective in their recording of details, though, the best physicians will keep their arguments open. They will judge between which of the available details are critical and which are spurious, but they will strive to reserve judgment about the final diagnosis.

Rather than jumping to a final, single diagnosis, physicians maintain a list of possible diagnoses, called a "differential diagnosis," or simply "differential," in physician-to-physician lingo. A physician uses a differential as an open-ended argument to slow down his drive toward judgment. A differential lists all diagnoses that could explain the group of findings so far. Groups of academic internists will often try to one-up each other by adding obscure diagnoses to the differential for a case under discussion.

While intended to include every possibility, a differential doesn't simply pile diagnoses or throw them into a bag. Differentials organize diagnoses into hierarchies. Hierarchical organization schemes for a differential usually include rankings such as how common, how dangerous, and how easily excluded each diagnosis is.

First, how common. Considering population frequencies, physicians often say, "Common things are common," or, "If you hear hoofbeats, think horses before you think zebras." The most common diagnoses are not exclusively present, but are most commonly present. With that in mind, common diagnoses will top the list but will not end the list, which must include more rare zebra-diagnoses as well.

Second, how dangerous, or how immediate. The tenth diagnosis on the list in terms of population likelihood may pose the most significant immediate danger to the patient's life or well-being. Physicians prioritize these dangerous diagnoses that require expeditious exclusion or confirmation. For example, many diagnoses can explain leg swelling in a post-operative patient. A blood clot ranks very low on the list of most common things, but grabs attention and will be ruled out first because it threatens the life and limb of the patient.

Third, ease of exclusion. Ranking diagnoses by ease of exclusion also applies to differentials. If a doctor can easily remove four of the five most common diagnoses by a simple examination maneuver or test, she may prioritize these.

The best differentials include not only an exhaustive list of ranked diagnoses but a plan or algorithm through which the differential will be narrowed down. This diagnostic algorithm is really a map that guides the patient and physician through the differential toward a treatment-worthy or resolved diagnosis.

From his first visit with Anna, Dr. Smith should have had both pelvis tumor and workers' comp-driven-malingering on his differential diagnosis, but he should have also included other possibilities. A typical differential for a symptom of low back pain ranks muscle strain at the top of the most common list.

Tumors and infections top the most dangerous list, but are not common. Tumors and infections also rank highly on the ease-of-exclusion priority list. If back pain lasts more than a few weeks, physicians usually order radiographs of the spine, which will show most tumors or serious infections as Anna's did. Had her physician's differential stayed open, Anna would have had that critical radiograph that made the correct diagnosis months earlier.

At some points, while traveling along a diagnostic algorithm, a physician faces a persistent list of potential remaining diagnoses, from which she usually picks the most common and tries treatments. These treatments are essentially diagnostic experiments, seeking response to treatment as a confirmation of diagnosis. This therapy-as-diagnostic-test thinking backs that initial waiting period of a few weeks before ordering the first radiograph for low back pain.

Because most back pain episodes from muscle strains will resolve within that time, the physician tries to see if that first treatment intervention of waiting will resolve the concern, stopping the algorithm in its tracks. The thinking goes, "If we try this and the problem goes away, then we don't even care what name goes on the diagnosis."

All differentials and their algorithms depend on clear, honest, and trusting communication between physician and patient. If either the physician or patient isn't on board, differentials and algorithms fall apart.

With these algorithms in mind, consider the care provided in the ERs and urgent care centers so popular in American health care. Physicians practicing in such settings cannot trust that a patient will follow a given algorithm through the differential to arrive at its successful conclusion because they will not personally see the patient through the algorithm. The ER physician works within a narrow opportunity in time to rule out the most dangerous items on the differential that he might more effectively eliminate with a follow-up visit a few days later.

This prompts the opposite of Anna's problem; ER and urgent care center physicians feel compelled to order too many tests, too early in the algorithm. They don't have time to test diagnoses by experimenting with simple interventions, such as waiting a day or two.

While ER physicians enjoy no time-extended relationship with patients to work patiently on diagnostic algorithms, mistrust and misjudgment cloud algorithms in other physician-patient relationships.

Anna's doctor saw many gray arrows pointing toward one diagnosis, the diagnosis of worker's compensation-related malingering.

He suspected that she had an agenda. As his mind closed on other diagnoses, he ignored the gray arrows pointing in those other directions and even began to see some gray arrows that were not actually there.

Once he passed judgment, he left no room for trust in this particular case. It took a significant worsening of her symptoms for him to get beyond his suspicion of an agenda, restart the algorithm back a few months, order a radiograph, and refer Anna to me.

Although I don't think Anna had an agenda, many do.

Unfortunately, even agenda-ed patients, at risk of doing harm to themselves from seeking and receiving too much medical care, can have real problems that require real interventions. How do we talk to them? How do we build enough trust with them to proceed down an algorithm?

Winning

Another patient came to my sarcoma clinic on referral from a back pain treatment center. This young man lauded his pain specialists as the best doctors he had ever had. They aggressively managed his pain. I am not convinced that this helped him a great deal, but he and I can agree to disagree.

He had received multiple surgeries to fuse the bones of his lumbar spine together. Other procedures had placed electrical nerve stimulators of varied types near the spinal nerve roots. When these had failed, the pain specialists turned to "minimally" invasive procedures to numb, then cut, then burn small sensory nerves near the spine. Through all the treatments and since, the pain specialists kept the patient on hefty doses of narcotics. These doses blunted his personal interactions with his family and kept him from driving.

The patient came to his clinic visit with me with a list of narcotics so long and doses so high that you or I would stop breathing if we took half of them in one day. Still, his back and legs pained Chris all the time. After his thigh pain had increased following the last nerve burning procedure, the pain physicians had ordered some radiographs of the femur, or thigh bone. An abnormality on the radiographs prompted an MRI and referral to my clinic. The MRI showed a large mass filling about one quarter of the femur. Most of it had the appearance of a benign entity called a non-ossifying fibroma, a tumor of scar-like tissue inside the bone. Our very experienced musculoskeletal radiologist felt that the appearance of parts of it suggested more aggressive behavior than would be typical for a non-ossifying fibroma.

Radiologists and pathologists communicate with other physicians almost entirely through these differentials we have discussed. The radiologist's differential for Chris' femur lesion included some frightening --- however unlikely --- diagnoses. The radiologist and I agreed upon an ideal plan of obtaining additional imaging in six weeks to see if the lesion had changed.

The radiologist warned me: "Kevin, if you biopsy it, you'll have to scrape the whole thing out. The parts that worry me are at its two ends."

"Yes. I hope we don't have to go there," I answered.

I meant by "have to go there" that some patients simply cannot cope with waiting for an answer, even when waiting is the best first step in a diagnostic algorithm. Chris and I discussed his situation at length. I nearly convinced him to wait the six weeks. He would go home to think about it.

Chris's wife called my office the next day in tears.

"He didn't sleep at all last night. He feels the pain is getting worse."

While I had no doubt that the worsening pain overnight derived more from over-thinking than from worsening of the tumor in the bone, I didn't know for certain what was going on in his femur. I expected that it wasn't cancer, but neither the radiologist nor I could be sure. Unfortunately, the pattern of his pain, which can often tell me a lot about tumors in bones, could not be helpful given his complicated pain history.

"Tell Chris to come in again this afternoon," I offered. "We can talk more about it."

Chris and his wife came in. I reviewed it all with him again. I reviewed at length the risks and pain involved in surgery and why I wanted him to wait instead of pursuing it.

After nearly two hours, we ended up right where we had started. He appreciated my advice, but simply could not handle not knowing for six more weeks. He trusted my algorithm, but he could not tolerate it. Could I trust that he actually appreciated how much pain my surgery might cause him and how much it probably wouldn't fix the thigh pain that was his primary symptom?

Chris insisted that he understood these certain detriments and uncertain benefits of doing the surgery, but he was determined.

Was it interactions like this that prompted all his prior surgical and procedural interventions on his spine? Were those pain doctors as reluctant as I felt? Was I about to contribute to this patient harming himself by seeking so many unnecessary surgeries and procedures? But then, maybe his femur had a real problem. That is the worst part of patients whose histories and decisions are difficult to trust. They still can have cancer and infections, fractures and heart attacks.

The next week found Chris in the operating room. I scraped half a liter of tissue out of his femur, including the entire lesion, packed the defect with bone graft, and stabilized his then-weakened femur with a plate and screws. It was all fairly smoothly accomplished. Other than the predictable difficulty of managing postoperative pain in a man whose body was already accustomed to high doses of narcotics, the entire episode of care avoided any untoward surprises. He recovered back to his baseline level of pain by about three months after surgery. He was no better. The pathology showed --- almost sadly --- an entity as uneventful as the surgery. The large, benign non-ossifying fibroma contained no features that raised concern for cancer.

I wished I hadn't done the biopsy.

Chris didn't. Despite the surgical pain, he and his wife both slept soundly for the latter half at least of those six weeks that would have been the wait for the next imaging.

I couldn't have communicated more with him. Could I have communicated better? Could I have listened better the first day or in the first twenty minutes of the second day and saved myself a couple of hours of time trying to convince them of another choice? Should I have refused to do the surgery? I wasn't sure it was the wrong thing to do; it was just the course of two potential diagnostic algorithms that I didn't prefer.

Chokehold

I have recently had a friend experience such decisions from the other side. Without addiction to prescription pain medications and without a history of seeking multiple painful, invasive interventions, she still faced decisions mired in diagnostic uncertainty.

Years before our families met, she had experienced Hodgkin's lymphoma as a teenager, managed successfully with chemotherapy and radiation. After a couple of disease-free decades, she began to notice energy loss and generalized weakening. This progressed over months. She brought it to my attention. I arranged for her to reinitiate care with a lymphoma specialist at my cancer institute.

The lymphoma specialist felt the lymph nodes in her neck were enlarged. The doctor ordered a CT scan of the neck to better evaluate their actual size. The radiologist didn't see any lymph nodes on the scan that were larger than the normal size. He did find a nodule on one side of the thyroid. We arranged for my friend to see an ear, nose and throat surgeon, also at my institute.

The surgeon performed a needle biopsy of the lesion. This showed thyroid cancer.

In all likelihood, the new cancer resulted from the radiation her neck had received two decades earlier. We will never know beyond doubt, but it remains the best guess. The surgeon recommended removal of the half of the thyroid that contained the nodule. The procedure would serve mostly diagnostic purposes, but would also end up providing the definitive treatment if the pathologist confirmed that they had "gotten it all."

The surgeon removed the diseased half of the thyroid without incident. My friend called me to discuss the new pathology report after she received the news. The nodule had been the more aggressive of the two common types of thyroid cancer.

"Kevin, what would you do?" she asked.

"I am certainly no expert in thyroid cancer. What did he tell you?"

"He said that the old school protocol would be to remove the rest of the thyroid, as this was the follicular type of thyroid cancer --- but he prefers not to. He said that he rarely if ever does remove the other half in cases like this. He thinks that is the direction that his entire field is shifting toward."

"Do you understand what is involved in removal of the entire thyroid?" I asked.

"Yes. He said that I will be certain to require life-long thyroid hormone replacement medications."

"That's right, you will."

"But if I don't take it out, I will simply hang where I am until either a future scan comes up positive or I make it for a few years with consistently negative scans."

"Yes. How unlikely did the surgeon think it would be that the other side has additional cancer?"

"Very unlikely, he thought. The margins were negative around the nodule itself, and it was no more than about four millimeters in size anyway. Kevin, I just can't imagine the waiting process all over again. I've already been through the whole cancer thing before, with the years of follow-up visits."

"Well, you will go through that follow-up again regardless of your current decision."

"True, but it just feels different to choose maybe to leave some cancer in me."

"In exchange for taking a not-so-bad pill daily for the rest of your life?"

"Yes. The life-long pill a day doesn't frighten me, the other possibility does."

"While I generally try to warn people against making decisions out of fear alone, I think you can phrase this another way. You have looked at two potential ways of managing this clinical situation. One will give you fairly definitive answers in the short-term, the other won't. I think you've made your decision."

Her surgeon protested some about going through with the second surgery. He met with her a couple of times. I think that may have served only to drill into me the parallel character of her experience to Chris's with me. She finally insisted on the removal of the rest of her thyroid. She and her surgeon proceeded.

In this third and final specimen, the pathologist found much more extensive presence of follicular thyroid carcinoma through the tissues and even abutting the capsule of the thyroid itself. It had grown in an infiltrative pattern, making it difficult to have visualized with the CT scan or the multiple thyroid ultrasounds my friend had received by this point.

This new diagnostic material, unwanted by the physician but insisted upon by the patient, increased the disease staging. Because of it, my friend then also underwent radioactive iodine treatments to eradicate any additional tumor that might have been present elsewhere in her body. No one really predicted it. Even my friend thought that she was asking for something beyond necessary.

We can only know the answers to the questions we ask diagnostically. We may not know those answers with great confidence, but we can be confidently ignorant of the results of every test we don't pursue.

In no way do I advocate that more diagnostic testing is better, or that the shotgun approach is more likely to hit the target. The best for which we can hope is that physicians and patients will communicate effectively, sharing their algorithm as it unfolds. In the end, my friend and her physician did this. Even though they disagreed on the ideal next step, they agreed to uphold the mutual trust and work together on their way down an algorithm.

Mistrust can cripple that algorithm. Mistrust develops when a physician believes a patient is either not interested in getting better or more interested in gaming the system. It also develops when a patient doesn't believe the physician has her best interests in mind. As mistrust poisons communication, the uncertainty strengthens. Most challenging is the fact that the uncertainty both engenders poor communication and is exacerbated by it. Because diagnosis requires guessing and trying and waiting for answers, physicians and patients must approach it as members of the same team, or both will lose the game.

Starting Your Conversation. . . .

Watching Ps and Qs

Principle: Miscommunication between patients and physicians escalates when trust is lacking.

Ask your physician: Will you please summarize or repeat back to me what you have heard from me?

Losing the Game

Principle: Some patients attempt to game the system. Some physicians suspect patients are gaming the system. Such suspicions worsen uncertainty.

Ask your physician: May I summarize what I have heard from you, to make sure that we are both on the same page?

Incongruity

Principle: Some physicians worry about telling patients that a diagnostic test found nothing when the patients have invested a lot emotionally into anticipation of an answer to their troubles.

Ask your physician: Are we pursuing this finding because you think it is the real answer to my problem or just because it is the only thing to pursue? Will you please tell me when we reach the point where you don't know?

The Last Shall be First

Principle: Physicians organize potential diagnoses for each patient according to how common, how dangerous, and how easily ruled out each is, then proceed down an algorithm hoping to arrive at a final diagnosis with the patient.

Ask your physician: Have we ruled out everything immediately dangerous? What else is on your list of possible diagnoses for my condition? What is next?

Winning

Principle: Some patients cannot tolerate waiting for an answer, which is often the safest route toward a diagnosis. Ultimately, physicians and patients must both feel comfortable with the approach.

Ask your physician: Would time, rather than another battery of tests, help us clarify my problem at this point? Will another month or a couple of weeks lose precious time in terms of missing some opportunity for treatment?

Chokehold

Principle: Peace of mind can figure powerfully into the decisions patients make on the way toward a diagnosis. Some prefer to tolerate great nuisance over minor ongoing risks.

Ask your physician: What next step gives me the surest bet for an answer? What next step minimally intrudes into my life and well-being?

Part Two: Treatment

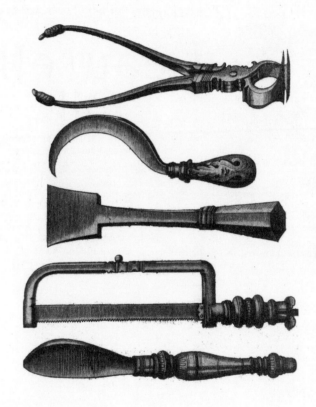

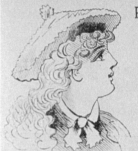

WIGGLE ROOM

Oil Slick

"You can drink it, or rub it on."

My friend detailed the conversation she had heard many times between a surgeon and the few patients for whom he could offer no surgery. Her sports orthopaedic surgery fellowship director offered surgery of some type to almost every patient whom he met in his clinic. These patients often travelled from the far reaches of the nation or even homes abroad to see him.

His aggressive approach satisfied patients, even if it shocked my friend at first. Apparently, to any patient for whom no surgery could be considered beneficial --- even at a stretch --- he offered what he called an "amino-salve" to help their aches, pains, or arthritis. The salve could be taken by mouth or applied directly to the sore joint. The surgeon personally developed the recipe and included in his pitch a testimonial that he used it himself daily.

As much as this surgeon's amino-salve sales pitch smacks of the snake oil salesmen of the old Wild West, it may be exactly what those patients need. He certainly remains very busy, and with a long-distance, high-society clientele. His patients are far from bereft of alternative options for orthopaedic knee care. I don't know if his salve works or not. No one does.

The uncertainty upon which the dishonest snake oil salesmen capitalized in the old Wild West was no different than what enabled their more reputable counterparts, the "real" physicians of the 19th century, to do even crazier things, like blood-letting. They may have performed these bleeding treatments with greater decorum, but were they any better? When we don't know, we try things.

It's a good thing, too. Without innovation and the gumption to try new things on the part of patients and physicians, we might have little more to offer than blood-letting or amputation.

Nonetheless, uncertainty remains rampant in treatment decisions.

Physicians deal with this uncertainty in very different ways. Some capitalize on it. Others run from it.

A hip surgeon I know inherited his prior partner's practice after the partner retired from surgery. In the few years leading up to retirement, this partner's wariness of surgery led him to great efforts to avoid it for his patients. Before he would replace a hip, his patient had to decline nearly to wheelchair-bound status.

Upon this senior partner's retirement, the younger surgeon built a backlog of many months' worth of cases as soon as he started seeing these long-postponed hip arthritis patients. Far from cavalier in the indication for hip surgery himself, he still felt embarrassed that his partner hadn't offered surgery to many of these patients earlier.

Most orthopaedic surgeons will fall somewhere between these two extremes. On one end there is surgery for almost everyone and if not surgery, amino-salve; on the other end there is the withholding of surgical intervention until patient symptoms become completely incapacitating. That said, moderation as one's solution doesn't change the principle. When we don't know the "correct" approach, decisions that must be made will require us to exercise judgment of some type.

The influence of physician preference is one common manifestation of uncertainty in medical treatments. The range can be broad.

We witness treatment uncertainty in yet unstudied clinical questions, yet poorly studied clinical questions, and clinical questions which have been studied, but showed no meaningful difference between two potential options. What to do in this last scenario, which is rather common, raises many ethical and economic questions. If two options, when compared, have no demonstrable difference, top-down administrated medical systems like HMOs and single-payer governmental health care programs will settle upon the cheapest option.

In most of the United States, where specific decisions have little bearing on costs to individuals, we see persistence of both options, dependent on physician and patient preferences. Some prefer the older of two options. This is usually cheaper. They consider it the tried and "true" option. Others prefer the latest, although not necessarily "greatest" option, which tends to be more expensive. Marketing to patients or physicians, potential conflicts of interest from physician-industry financial relationships, and many other messy factors weigh-in to these complex decisions. Again, the alternate answers physicians propose to these uncertainties on a case-by-case basis are not good or bad medicine, they are just different. We either don't know --- or potentially will never know --- a meaningful difference between the two.

Examples of these indistinguishable-benefit options are manifold in medicine. There are many options in each class of cholesterol medications, or blood-pressure medications, or brands of total knee implants. Rarely will a study compare two options in the same class head-to-head.

In fact, the rates at which physicians select a given option among the variety of seemingly equivalent options rarely matches a principled aim at either cost reduction or research-derived evidence. For example, Lipitor (atorvastatin) reigned for many years as the most prescribed of the varied and sundry statin-type cholesterol medications available.[1] Was it the oldest? No. Was it the cheapest? No. Was it backed by the greatest research track record? Not really. It *was* the most aggressively marketed. Is there anything medically wrong with this fact? No, but it illustrates that what decisions physicians and patients make within the undefined space of medical uncertainty will see the influence of many factors.

Are we certain that Lipitor doesn't differ from other statins? No. Nor will we ever be, most likely.

Principle and Interest

In addition to the fact that drug companies have no incentive to test their drugs against each other, the vagaries of treatment uncertainty muddle the evaluation of any intervention in medicine. The placebo effect contributes heavily to this muddle.[2] It merits some discussion here. Physicians and scientists have written volumes about the placebo effect in medical and experimental science literature.

You are doubtless aware of the basic premise. When a trial tests a new drug in a placebo-controlled fashion, the group of patients not receiving the investigational drug receives instead a "placebo," or fake treatment, which neither the patient nor the physician can distinguish from the investigational drug. That last bit we call double-blinding. Placebos simply enable the researchers to control as many variables as possible in the experiment. The use of placebos recognizes that patient and physician perceptions can powerfully skew results if not controlled, or equalized between the different groups.

The world of medicine discusses the magnitude of these placebo effects far less frequently. A placebo group is necessary as a control because surprisingly large portions of the studied population, just by thinking that they are receiving a remedy, will experience an improvement in their symptoms, better disease management, and even increases in side effects. The size of the placebo effect has no known standards, or it would just be added as an adjustment to any trial of a new drug. Generally speaking, more drastic interventions typically generate larger placebo effects. The few times they have been used in trials, placebo-surgery groups have recorded high-magnitude effects, usually in the 30- to 40-percent range.

One of my professors repeatedly taught that nothing makes the results in a surgical series look worse than long-term follow-up, but nothing makes them look better than the lack of a control group. With no placebo-blinded control, one can erroneously attribute all the measurably good results of an intervention to that intervention. Really, some large portion of the measurably good results is better attributed to the patient's perception that an intervention took place.

A few years ago, an orthopaedic team at a veteran's hospital in Texas performed a research study with a sham-surgery placebo group.[3] The results shocked the world of orthopaedic surgery --- or did they? Patients with mild to moderate osteoarthritis of the knee were randomized to arthroscopic debridement (cleaning out using instruments placed into the knee through small incisions), arthroscopic irrigation (washing of liters of saline through the knee, via similar incisions, but without the use of instruments to remove degenerated tissues), or sham surgery, in which the small incisions were made, but only through the skin, not all the way through to the knee. Patients didn't know which surgery they had received. Even the sham surgery patients heard lots of fluid splashing around in the operating room. Using patient questionnaires to assess outcomes in terms of pain and function, the study found no difference between the groups at one year after surgery. So all of the benefit perceived by the surgeons who had been offering this intervention to patients may have been no more than the placebo effect of offering a surgery!

More interesting is the medical community's response to this study. It confirmed the long-held suspicion among conservative-minded surgeons that arthroscopic clean-outs provide no helpful benefit as a treatment for arthritis and should not be offered. In the year or so after the publication of this paper, the number of these purportedly unnecessary surgeries dropped dramatically. If an intervention such as this, with its inherent risks and costs, provided no meaningful benefit, no one should pursue it, right? Well, maybe. If there is no difference in outcome between groups, it must not be hurting patients either, correct? So, maybe, anything goes.

If a physician convinces herself that she has seen some patients helped by it, and convinces patients that they may be in that sub-group of the overall population, maybe it is okay. No harm done, at least, right? Likely following this type of thinking, the rate of arthroscopic debridement for osteoarthritis of the knee began to rise again after a year or two of reduction in cases.

It would be easy for me to condemn this practice as money-driven and mercenary silencing or ignorance of the evidence, but that wouldn't be entirely fair. I know of salaried surgeons who receive no incremental remuneration for specific case performance who still offer this option to some patients. I know of one orthopaedic surgeon who requested the arthroscopic debridement for his own knee.

When we don't know, we don't know. Even if it is only placebo effect, how else can a knee surgeon achieve a surgery-sized placebo effect for his patient?

Bucking

The issue of conflicting interests stands paramount when we become aware of how much opinion and preference impact treatment decisions. Another treatment decision, how to surgically repair a certain type of hip fracture, exposes some of these.

Clinical trials have rigorously compared two treatment options for these hip fractures, plate-and-screw implants or intramedullary nail and screw implants.[4] Trials comparing the first generation of the intramedullary devices didn't fare well against the older, cheaper plate devices, due to complications. Later versions of the intramedullary devices corrected some of these design flaws. Comparison trials of the later generation intramedullary devices found no demonstrable difference from the old standard plate devices.

So, anything goes, right? Maybe some surgeons perform one better than the other? Shouldn't the surgeon use the one with which she performs the best? Well, it turns out that the more expensive intramedullary devices also bill a higher surgical fee. In America, surgeons fix a majority of these fractures with these more expensive and higher-billing devices. In the United Kingdom and Europe, where implant budgets are capped, surgeons utilize the cheaper plate devices almost exclusively.

Do I know that reimbursement patterns alone make these decisions?

Of course not. But I have a sneaking suspicion. Remember, though, that the money argument can be made against either decision. The European bureaucrats, trying to save a buck, choose the cheaper implant for the systems they control. The American surgeons, trying to make a buck, choose the more expensive implant that also gets them a higher surgical fee. The independent, slightly rebellious part of me applauds the American surgeons who choose the cheaper plate implant and the European surgeons who insist on using the nail.

I cannot fairly judge even the physicians who let finances influence their decisions as making those decisions with *only* finances in mind. Most have no intention to hurt patients to make a buck. They don't choose bad options because of money, usually. They simply allow money to help divide the gray into black and white, when no more noble force seems to divide it for them. Uncertainty opens multiple paths, none of which has been determined to be clearly better or worse than the others. Financial pressures usually only direct which among the uncertain paths is chosen.

Mind the Gap

Most graduating medical students take the Hippocratic oath in some form or another as they receive their medical degrees. Nearly all forms of the oath contain a promise to benefit patients and "first do no harm." Clearly, this represents an ethical promise to *intend* no harm through care provided to patients. Beyond intention itself, this promise could never hold up. The Institute of Medicine's report, "To Err is Human" brought critical focus to the issue of errors in medicine in 1999.[5] There has been plentiful press coverage and much public discourse about the many patients whom errors in medicine have injured or killed, ever since.

No mistake need be made for a patient to be harmed by the tests and treatments administered by physicians. After we lock up the very few physicians *intending* to harm and account for the basic rates of error to which all human systems are prone, medicine will hurt many more patients simply by their falling outside of the hoped-for effects of appropriate treatments. Every treatment and most tests usher in side effects, to be sure. Most also simply fail to achieve their stated goals in a given portion of patients to whom they are applied. This explains the great difficulty we encounter in comparing different treatments. It explains how the sandbox of treatment uncertainty grew into such a large play space.

Consider some of the things that we know we don't know. For example, for sickle cell anemia, in spite of our ability to diagnose it with single-DNA-base-pair precision, we offer no cure.[6] We don't even know what initiates or how to quell the crises to which patients with sickle cell anemia are dangerously prone. We have understood its genetics for many decades but stand no closer to knowing effective treatments for this challenging disease than we did fifty years ago.

Physicians have taken the Hippocratic oath since the ancient Greeks, but in the days prior to the Second World War, what physicians didn't know certainly did hurt their patients. As medical technology progressed across the last century, we began to know enough at least to net positive on the benefit/harm balance sheet. But what do we know? And what does knowing mean to a physician?

Gaps in evidence-based medical know-how are plentiful. They far exceed the filled-in areas. Physicians don't simply throw up their hands and do nothing. They should not capitulate so easily. Instead, they fill in these gaps with decisions.

Physician preference and patient preference and payer preference all impinge upon those decisions, but even when we remove preference and financial pressures, we retain the gaps in need of filler. We don't send patients experiencing a sickle cell anemia crisis back home to suffer alone. We do something.

Physicians often fill in gaps in treatment certainty with physiologic reasoning. By physiologic reasoning, I mean the process of making an educated guess as to the effects of an intervention based on an understanding of the biological pathway it is designed to affect, but an absence of large population-based randomized, controlled trials of the intervention itself.

Physiologic reasoning figures prominently in medical thinking. Some of it simply applies common sense. If a bone is broken and crooked, physicians have observed that it will usually heal in the crooked position. This phenomenon is *observed* physiology. Straighten it, and hold it in a straightened position, and it will heal in a straight position. This is *applied* physiology.

As another example, the human body increases the heart rate in response to danger or need of additional oxygen in the tissues. It accomplishes this elevated heart rate by an increase of adrenaline signaling to beta-adrenergic receptors in the heart.

Beta-blockers are a class of medications that interrupt this signal. The interruption of this signal physiologically lowers heart rate as well as lowering the acceleration of the heart rate in response to such stimuli. For conditions in which physicians consider an elevated heart rate dangerous, they have reasoned that beta-blockers will reduce this danger.

Not all physiology is as straightforward as the mechanical aspects of bone healing or the heart-rate reduction achieved by pharmaceutical beta-blockade. Not all physiology is as easily manipulated either.

These limits seriously challenge physiologic reasoning as our navigator through the fog of treatment uncertainty. We base the predictions made by physiologic reasoning on an incomplete understanding of the potential effects of the intervention in something as complex as the human body.

For example, beta-blockers are sometimes --- but not always --- a good method of reducing high blood pressure. For some patients their high blood pressure results more from other inputs than those addressed by beta-blockers. Furthermore, beta-blockers have unwanted effects beyond the heart rate and blood pressure, like an increase in the rate of depression among those medicated with them. The system has additional inputs, additional read-outs.

Despite these complexities in physiology, physicians set their minds to thinking about what makes the most rational sense when they have no better information to go on. The educated guesses that result may be better than uneducated guesses.

I think they are.

They are nonetheless *guesses*, though.

Physicians would be wise to remember this point.

We would be even wiser, I think, to explain this point to our patients, when our counsel impacts their decisions.

New Flash

When one considers the complexity of human biology, the fact that many physiologically reasoned interventions have proven dead wrong when applied in a population and actually measured should not surprise. We find a perfect example in the use of oral estrogen pills for peri- and post-menopausal women, called hormone replacement therapy (HRT). The story of the rise of HRT and its subsequent near disappearance over the last decade is one of the most public debacles in modern medicine.

Physicians made a number of observations concerning peri- and post-menopausal physiology over the years. Uncomfortable hot flashes, mood swings, osteoporosis (severely declined bone density), risk of heart attack, and the rates of some cancers rise abruptly as an aging woman's ovaries stop their production of estrogen hormones. Physicians therefore reasoned --- quite logically at first glance --- that avoidance of the decline in circulating estrogen hormone levels was desirable. Replacing them with a medication would avoid the abrupt onset of hot flashes and increases in risks for mood swings, heart disease, strokes, cancer, and osteoporosis. So confident were physicians in the benefits of this intervention, based on a few small studies and a lot of physiologic reasoning, that they considered it the standard of care, even for women not troubled by the uncomfortable hot flashes and mood swings of the peri-menopausal period.

In the 1990s, astonishing numbers of peri- and post-menopausal women took hormone replacement therapy. It was the magic medicine that made you feel better, avoid mood swings, and even lower your risk of osteoporosis, heart disease, stroke, and cancer. Sound too good to be true? Well, it was.

I make no argument that physicians were deceptive or dishonest in any way as they prescribed these medications. They were practicing the standard of care. They were not in "error." Quite the contrary, physicians who didn't offer their patients hormone replacement therapy were criticized as behind-the-times and not practicing the evidence-based standard of care.

Enter: The Women's Health Initiative.[7] This large, prospective, randomized, controlled study discovered that when you actually measure rates of heart disease and stroke and breast cancer in populations of women using hormone replacement therapy, they go up, not down. The world of medicine, utterly ashamed at the product of its physiologic reasoning, then backtracked rapidly. Three years after the realization, it was rare to find any woman still taking hormone replacement therapy.

One disease in particular became a bigger challenge in the wake of the HRT debacle. Estrogen hormone supplementation effectively prevented and treated post-menopausal osteoporosis. In the wake of the Women's Health Initiative reports, physicians have been leery of hormone replacement therapy (perhaps more out of embarrassment than the fear of the real level of risks) even for this disease for which it worked beautifully.

They began to grasp around for alternative options for managing osteoporosis. Only one group of agents even approached the success of hormone replacement therapy in maintaining bone density: bisphosphonates.[8] Bisphosphonates mimic and incorporate into the bone mineral and then inhibit the normal, slow destruction of bone.

A bit of physiologic reasoning comes into play with bisphosphonates as well. A normal, baseline level of bone destruction constantly erodes the mineral density in the skeleton. A tandem process of bone production matches this very closely. The two processes work together continuously to replace or "turnover" the skeleton. This bone turnover critically rids the skeleton of micro-cracks and other damage from the usual wear and tear. The disease process of osteoporosis uncouples the two sides of bone turnover, resulting in bone production that fails to maintain balance with the destruction. Hormone replacement tends to re-balance, or even over-balance in the good direction, the coupling of this bone turnover. Bisphosphonates, on the other hand, simply slow or halt the destruction half of it.

Despite the lack of long-term experience with bisphosphonates at the time, they became the go-to drugs for osteoporosis in the wake of the fading use of HRT. That makes physiologic sense, right? They stop the bone turnover, the primary disease process in osteoporosis.

Just like hormone replacement therapy, bisphosphonates certainly increase the mineral density of bones. Mineral density of bone previously proved to predict fracture risk with reasonable precision. But what happens when you stop the repair and replacement of micro-cracks for multiple years?

Unfortunately, we didn't reason quite that far ahead of ourselves. An increasing number of older women now sustain seemingly inexplicable femur shaft fractures after years of bisphosphonate therapy. Notably, femur shaft fractures don't typically associate with osteoporosis itself. Will we backtrack again? I don't know yet. Clearly, our physiologic reasoning fills in gaps in knowledge only as far as the depth, accuracy, and --- now we know --- duration of the understanding we have and hope to exploit.

The hormone-replacement-therapy debacle also teaches us that the results of studies that gather the most correct and useful data can take a long time. Usually, we are too cheap and too impatient to pay and wait for the correct data before implementing the idea on a broad scale.

That physicians want to provide solutions to health concerns helped create the hormone-replacement-therapy problem. Patients also want them. Sometimes wanting solutions leads us to jump with both feet into water that our toes have not touched long enough to ascertain its temperature. These are not evil desires on either the physicians' or the patients' part. Dangerously, though, we sometimes presume more than we actually know. At these moments, uncertainty can really get the best of us.

Guilt

Another controversial response to data came from the press release of the *story* of a trial's results preceding the publication of the *actual data* in the medical literature. The National Acute Spinal Cord Injury Study (NASCIS) comprised a series of three large multi-institutional trials testing a variety of steroid dosing protocols in the setting of traumatic spinal cord injuries.[9]

The use of steroids in the setting of spinal cord injury derived initially from physiologic reasoning that the inflammation arising after traumatic injury will damage the spinal cord beyond the injury itself. Reasoning therefore inspired the use of steroids, the most potent anti-inflammatory pharmaceuticals we have. Researchers had amplified this physiologic reasoning by indexing a variety of protective effects by using steroids in animal models of spinal cord injury. The NASCIS trials attempted to bring this reasoning and animal data to the benefit of patients on a large scale.

Spinal cord injuries devastate the individuals and families affected by them. Unlike the life-changing diagnoses with which I deal regularly in the world of cancer, spinal cord injuries don't give patients any time to settle into the idea that life will never be the same. In a moment, life changes permanently. Traumatic spinal cord injuries primarily strike a young, male and active population, exactly the population most emotionally fragile with regard to physical disability, which arrives suddenly, severely, and irreversibly in most spinal cord injuries.

Some spinal cord injuries result from a momentary foolish decision on the patient's part. He may have dived into a shallow river or driven a motorcycle too quickly around a curve. He may have attempted rock climbing without harness or ropes on a too-difficult pitch. Such circumstances taint the emotional experience of a spinal cord injury with even more bitterness. The individual often will have ahead of him years or decades of sitting, pondering his momentary lapse in judgment, heaping guilt and anger on top of the mourning for his former life.

I have personally cared for a few of these severe traumatic spinal cord injury patients during my training. Anyone who has witnessed these situations acutely, or seen their final outcomes, would share the general sense of desperation to improve our treatment for these injuries.

Nerves in the central nervous system, or the brain and spinal cord, cannot take a joke. These tissues have virtually no regenerative potential in adults. This means that whatever function an injury steals will not return. There are few (and they are miraculous) stories of recovery of spinal cord functions that have been lost from physical injury to the tissue itself.

All these factors --- the irreversibility of any lost motor and sensory function, the crushing life effects of such impairments, the suddenness of the change, the youth of the victims --- charge the decision-making involved in emergency care of these patients with powerful emotions.

When the study coordinators of NASCIS II felt that they had important positive findings to report, they didn't want to wait for the medical publication circuit to run its bureaucratic gauntlet. The popular media released the story weeks before the *New England Journal of Medicine* published the full scientific paper. Unfortunately, this led patients, patient families and care providers to seek to pursue treatments, the data behind which the providers hadn't yet fully evaluated. This was problem number one. Unfortunately, early release of the story prior to the data wasn't the only problem with NASCIS II.

Taken at face value, NASCIS II found no difference in results between the treatment groups, including one placebo group, one steroid group, and one group receiving another type of drug. The authors didn't promote *that* story. Negative stories never receive much attention. With a negative primary result, the statisticians proceeded to secondary analyses, which ultimately pared the groups down to about 30 percent of overall study population. Between some of these pared-down groups, subtle differences were identified; these provided the punch line for which everyone hoped. Even the subtle advantages NASCIS II reported from steroid therapy offered to specific sub-groups of spinal cord injury patients have had difficulty standing the test of time since.

As physicians around the world applied the steroid treatments promoted by the trial more widely, they identified alarming rates of bad side effects. In retrospect, it came to light that the study hadn't recorded side effects as diligently as it had recorded spinal cord function. Further, when looked at honestly, even the study's primary report claimed no *lasting* benefit of the intervention for spinal cord function; the benefits perceived in treated patients during early recovery didn't persist at the outcome assessment of the same patients one year after the injury.

Don't misunderstand me. I have no reason to believe that any of these investigators was trying to pull the wool over anyone's eyes. I am not personally aware of any financial conflicts of interest that would have swayed them. An independent NIH-appointed panel rigorously oversaw the massive project beyond even the investigators themselves.

Sometimes we want an improvement to our status quo so badly, and we feel so much confidence that the physiologic reasoning leads us toward such improvement, that we will squint our eyes while looking at it long enough to imagine the fuzzy outlines of improvement when none may be there.

Vigorous Precision

Another such wishful-thinking, physiologically-reasoned advance in medicine flourished and fizzled to an amplitude similar to hormone replacement therapy, but in a much faster course from beginning to top and then back to bottom.

Non-steroidal anti-inflammatory drugs, or NSAIDs (pronounced, "én-seds"), directly inhibit the function of an enzyme involved in the chemical pathway that initiates inflammation. You are familiar with these drugs as ibuprofen (trade name Advil), naproxen (trade name Aleve), and many other prescription varieties. These have been available for decades. There are known side effects to these drugs as a class. One may not correctly call the morbidity of these drugs "side effects" at all. Rather, the *expected effects* of the drug have some desirable and some less desirable results in human physiology. Specifically, these drugs inhibit an enzyme called cyclo-oxygenase (COX), halting a tissue's recruitment of additional inflammatory cells, which otherwise would accumulate around its active chemical pathway.

COX enzymes play a role in inflammation, but also in clotting of blood in arteries and protecting the lining of the stomach. Physicians have used the fact that NSAIDs inhibit blood clotting as one means of preventing some heart attacks in at-risk patients. Not surprisingly, stomach ulcers are the most common adverse effects from NSAID treatments. We use NSAIDs commonly enough that these stomach ulcers became a major public health problem. Even at the height of the AIDS epidemic in the United States, more people died yearly from bleeding ulcers secondary to NSAID use than died of AIDS and its related infections. This background drove a strong --- even if less emotionally charged --- desire to improve the status quo.

Scientists discovered in the late 1980s that humans carry two versions of the COX enzyme. Critically, the second type functions in inflammation and the first in protecting the stomach and slowing clot formation.

What if a drug could inhibit only the second type? That question was pursued vigorously by a number of large pharmaceutical companies. Their efforts bore fruit. Rofecoxib (trade name Vioxx) and celecoxib (trade name Celebrex) hit the drug market with as big a bang (and bigger bucks) as any new drug in my memory. Both promised the pain relief of NSAIDs without the stomach ulcers. To doctors, they advertised that the ulcers would be less of a problem; to patients, they suggested these drugs would generate less stomach upset (much more common and usually not related to the dangerous ulcers physicians worry about).

Some appropriately large, randomized, placebo-controlled trials were organized on the drugs' path toward the market.[10] All of them bore spiffy names like the VIGOR trial and the PRECISION trial. The specificity of the drugs for cyclo-oxygenase 2 (also called COX-2) alone proved weaker in humans than they may have hoped. Nonetheless, the story sold well.

Again, the drug companies pitched COX-2 inhibitors to physicians with the promise that this would extend the possibility of NSAID use to more frail patients who could not tolerate or even risk intestinal bleeds. Unfortunately, some such patients still developed dangerous ulcers on COX-2 selective inhibitors.

Specifically, one of the trials noticed that if a patient took even a baby aspirin daily to protect the heart, the addition of Vioxx no longer spared any of the stomach and intestinal NSAID effects. This, of course, reduced the potentially treatable population; there are few over 65 who don't take a daily baby aspirin for their heart.

Although neither as perfect nor as trouble-free as hoped for, COX-2 selective inhibitors still somewhat accomplished their stated medical goals. They unequivocally accomplished the companies' business goals with wild success as they flooded the market. So why the fall? Why have their sales plummeted from the initial bang? Why was one even pulled from the market?

Ironically enough, in the case of these selective cyclo-oxygenase inhibitors, the physiologic reasoning could have proffered all the risks up-front, if only we had undertaken complete physiologic reasoning from the known facts. As I mentioned, few people over 65 don't take a daily baby aspirin to thin the ability of their platelets to clot in their arteries. Clotting in arteries most commonly causes heart attacks and strokes. Most people over 65 need their blood thinned in this way because it actually works to prevent these heart attacks and strokes.

The big problem that arose in careful review of one of the large trials was that patients receiving standard NSAIDS that hit both types of COX enzymes rather than selectively the second type only, had fewer heart attacks. The company pulled Vioxx from the market as an un-safe drug. I am not convinced of any great loss to society in Vioxx's demise, but it illustrates the point. Physicians could have reasoned physiologically that increased blood clotting would result from drugs that didn't stop the COX enzymes involved in blood clotting. Medicine didn't extend its initial reasoning to this appropriate conclusion. It stopped after reaching the conclusion it wanted to see.

Even when physiologic reasoning *can* provide relatively complete answers to a given area of uncertainty, it cannot escape its fundamental character as *reasoning*. Bias can corrupt reasoning. If one wants a specific result from the exercise of reason, he is much more likely to obtain that result. That bias may arise from a drug manufacturer trying to make a buck (or a few billion) or a physician or patient seriously wanting a solution to a clinical problem. Either bias can seriously cloud reason, introducing flaws, elevating uncertainty.

The Upper Crust

We all want solutions that work. Sometimes, when we have developed a solution that basically works for a problem, we want to stop looking at it critically. Uncertainty creeps in whether we pay attention or not, but most ominously when our vigilance relaxes. Such unacknowledged uncertainty haunts the history of coronary artery bypass graft (CABG, pronounced "cabbage") surgery, the open-chest surgeries performed to re-vascularize the heart. Heart surgeons undertake CABG after identifying a heart attack or a critically narrowed vessel that fails to provide adequate blood flow to the heart muscle itself. CABG surgery has saved or extended as many or more lives as any surgery out there.

In rankings of the most life-changing interventions available in all of modern medicine, CABG surgery often tops the list. The surgeons who perform CABG in community or academic medical centers very rarely do anything but these highly specialized surgeries. The development of successful CABG surgery required much more than the training of a cadre of nimble-fingered surgeons. It required the development of technology that provided temporary oxygenation and pumping of blood while these surgeons worked on the heart. Indeed, the development of this bypass pump technology defined the medical centers that pioneered open-heart surgery of any kind in the 1950s and 60s.

To some great extent, the early successes of CABG surgery achieved miracle status. CABG provided a cure for what had been a wholly incurable problem. More than any other surgery, perhaps, physicians have subjected CABG to a number of randomized controlled trials, most demonstrating its gold standard efficacy in restoring health to diseased heart muscle. Despite the real risks of peri-operative mortality, this procedure truly saves lives. Where is the uncertainty in that, right? We know this as we know all things in medicine, by populations rather than by individuals, but everything we looked at with this surgery appeared to favor it strongly for populations in need.

Over the years, the experience with CABG grew. It became more widely practiced and more evidence-based scientifically.

Uncertainty met CABG less in ORs, clinics or trial databases and more in the OR locker rooms and doctors' lounges of hospitals where surgeons performed it.

In these places, physicians began to bandy about a term to describe some specific results of CABG. The term's casual, almost slang character befitted such clandestine settings. I doubt, though, any uttered it casually at all, or in any but the most hushed, private, hoping-it-was-not-truth tones. The term didn't initially reach the stature of public discourse. How could one rightly discuss "pump head" with the public when no one was really sure if the phenomenon it described was fact or fiction? Right?

Nonetheless, it troubled physicians. "Pump head" described the phenomenon of open-heart surgery knocking the upper crust off of patients' mental status.[11] Some patients woke up from heart bypass and CABG or some other structural surgery on the heart slightly less there mentally than they were pre-operatively. At least they woke up, surgeons would comfort themselves, appropriately acknowledging that the surgery saved lives. This comfort didn't permanently assuage their conscience on the matter.

Eventually the heart team at Duke University decided to measure pump head, or the detectable changes in mental status that seemed to occur around surgery. It turns out that a majority of patients who go on heart bypass end up with at least 20 percent loss of measurable mental function. The first study remains one of the only large-scale studies of this phenomenon. Not surprisingly, medicine has now redubbed pump head as "post-perfusion syndrome." Someone in an OR locker-room somewhere must have thought "pump head" a little too brash or, perhaps, a little too clear to the uneducated ear.

Once again, I have to step back far enough to mention that I don't intend to slam heart surgery in general or CABG in specific. The challenge isn't that CABG should not be performed; the challenge is that because no one dared to look pump head directly in the face for so long, this uncertainty persisted unacknowledged for decades. We know little more now, even though we can discuss it in polite circles. Many argue that individuals with aggressive vascular disease (the type of patients receiving CABG surgeries) may be prone to the micro-strokes that we think cause post-perfusion syndrome. They argue that part of pump head is the natural course of the underlying disease process, rather than a complication of treatment. Some centers have started trying to perform CABG without connecting the heart to a bypass machine, an even more technically difficult feat. So far, studies have suggested that the bypass machine itself may not be the problem, but time will tell.

Perhaps less invasive methods that use technologically improved stents will eventually avoid the necessity of CABG altogether. Where the story will lead remains uncertain. Nonetheless, now that we can speak of these mental side effects of heart surgery and think about them, we can begin to understand them and hopefully educate our patients better about the decisions they face.

I admit that in my own field of orthopaedic surgery, some quietly wonder about the mental effects of anaesthesia for any reason in the elderly, and even more about procedures such as total joint arthroplasty that shower the lungs with small marrow fragments. Might a more subtle pump-head-like phenomenon hover beneath our notice in other fields? We only discover the treatment uncertainties that we dare to investigate. We usually only investigate the uncertainties that we publicly admit may exist.

The End Result

Physicians may fear such disclosures because public admission of medicine's weaknesses doesn't always go well for the one disclosing. (We shall see what people think of me after reading this book!) While new awareness of unpleasant truths is unpleasant, the dislike for these exposures touches another nerve as well. It suggests that people may not have recognized something that was directly impacting them. It is uncomfortable to feel that you have been duped, that you may have missed something.

The public often boldly insists that it knows medical quality when it sees it. I often laugh to myself when people tell me they have consulted a certain surgeon who did some famous athlete's surgery or that they saw Dr. So-and-So, who is the best total knee guy in town. How do they know? I cannot honestly comment on the quality of skills of even any of my partners in my department, let alone any colleagues in my community or beyond. These well-sold providers may be superlative in their skill, but I seriously doubt it. More likely, these physicians exploit the shrouded unknowns of medicine for their own gain. They may have an excellent business model, but very likely provide no truly superlative care.

Ernest Amory Codman was a surgeon at Massachusetts General Hospital and a professor at Harvard Medical School in the early 1900s. He suggested that we evaluate health interventions, either surgical or medical, by the end-result they produced in patient recipients.[12] He called it the "end-result concept." Although this thinking now pragmatically and philosophically guides most medical decision-making, the experts considered it heresy at the time. As he began to review the end-results of many of the interventions provided by his colleagues at the university, the results painted a less-than-glowing picture of their practiced standard of care. So unpopular were the reports he began to produce that his partners barred him from collecting such data. The end-result of his end-result concept was his getting kicked off the faculty and having his surgical privileges revoked.

Incensed, Dr. Codman fought back. In retort, he published an editorial cartoon in the *Boston Globe*. This cartoon depicted the rich Back Bay patient population as an ostrich, head-in-sand, offering Harvard its golden egg of patronage and business, despite complete lack of awareness of the end-results of the care it received. The response of his prior colleagues to the threat of his continued exposure of their faults doesn't surprise. The public response to his cartoon astonishes me.

Codman's honest, albeit taunting, exposure of the public's blind support of the Harvard medical faculty only expanded the outrage against him beyond the university's walls to the public. How dare he suggest that they blindly trusted the physicians and surgeons of Harvard? They *knew* how wonderfully Harvard physicians cared for them.

Although he published the cartoon out of anger, his assertion within it didn't miss the mark. He had collected enough data to

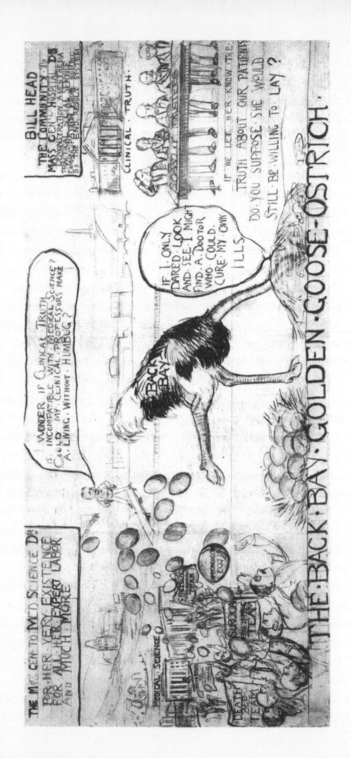

know that much of the care provided achieved no result with real value to the patients. Nonetheless, his honesty brought Dr. Codman into such public discredit that his career might have ended completely had it not been for a military assignment removing him from the fray.

The new assignment also gave him a separate venue in which to put his end-result concept to practice, far from the ire of the angry Bostonian clientele. While he never returned to prominence, Codman was eventually vindicated by the ultimate end-result of his ideas: outcomes now guide most decisions in medicine. Even the Harvard physicians realized they had been dead wrong in opposing him. That said, they never really mentioned this to their supportive patients.

Today people feel, perhaps no less erroneously, that they can identify the excellent medical practitioners in their community and beyond. They place elevated trust in certain physicians and health provider organizations for many reasons, but even today it is rarely due to measurably better care provided. People are just sure that they know medical quality when they see it, as were the Back Bay Bostonians.

We have all seen people blindly place their trust. Beyond medicine, in politicians, entertainers, military leaders, even business executives, success in garnering the support of followers has as much (or more) to do with apparent confidence as it does with effective policy ideas, remarkable performance talent, well-engineered strategic plans, or efficient management structures. Some politicians have mastered the art of saying with confidence what is far from the truth. Stated loudly, often, consistently, and confidently enough, many half-truths or even frank lies have become apparent truth in the eyes of followers.

We can argue about what exploitation of geopolitical uncertainties may or may not have done for our society, but medical uncertainty is quite different. Uncertainty in medical treatments is intimately personal. This intimacy promotes and perpetuates the uncertainty itself. Media will never probe into or expose the uncertainties undisclosed or even exploited by physicians as they speak to patients. Physician-patient conversations are private, both legally and ethically. Rarely will a patient even get the opinion of a second physician on a problem due to unhappiness with a first. What drives the trust in this private, blind, but surprisingly successful relationship between doctor and patient? I have no idea. I do believe that trust is at the core.

The breadth and depth of medically related knowledge continue to widen beyond the capacity of the human brain to comprehend. Simultaneously, the skill of computers to interact intelligently with complex data sets continues to expand. Naturally, some broach a dubious discussion of the role of human physicians in the future of medicine. Oft cited reasons for that role include the warm hand, the empathetic intellect, and the compassionate face. I don't agree with the necessity of these characteristics. I have seen many very successful physicians with none of the above. The human contribution to medicine may have much more to do with trust than it has to do with warmth, compassion, or empathy.

Physicians can be variably skilled at inviting patients into that vacant space of uncertainty in treatment. A patient can only enter it by investing a modicum of trust. Once inside with the patient, the physician may know more or less that what he offers can truly help the patient. Everyone outside that space will quite necessarily know less. Will the patient be trusted by the physician? Can the patient be trusted to learn what is known and not known?

Where it Hurts

Sometimes the failure of the medical community to communicate the rampant uncertainty in the practice of medicine comes back to bite it. Dr. Goldstein practices emergency medicine at a medium-sized community hospital in the suburbs of a major metropolitan city in the United States. He covers about 12 ER shifts each month but enjoys little leisure time in between these. Dr. Goldstein performs another, arguably more difficult, job on his "off-service" days.

Attorneys hire Dr. Goldstein to help defend physicians sued for malpractice. On the stand, Dr. Goldstein strives to convince

juries that even though physicians may have missed or misman-
aged a plaintiff's diagnosis, the mistakes may derive from poor luck
rather than actual negligence or error on the part of the treating
physician. Defense attorneys certainly pay Dr. Goldstein for these
appearances in court. That said, he doesn't involve himself in this
work motivated by the money alone.

It frustrates Dr. Goldstein that some trial lawyers and the
patient-plaintiffs they represent exploit the natural uncertainties
of medicine as evidence of malpractice. He finds most challenging
in his role as a witness the explanation to juries of exactly how
uncertain so many things are in medicine.

Why is it so hard for people to see the rampant uncertainty that
physicians and patients leap into every time they enter clinics and
hospitals?

I believe that physicians have partly created this difficulty by
keeping uncertainty hidden. We leave unspoken too many doubts
and misgivings, leading the public to build false confidence in our
ability to control outcomes. Because we leave these uncertainties
hidden, we must swing wildly away from treatments we previously
recommended as soon as new data suggests that our initial enthusiasm was misdirected. The HRT, NASCIS, and COX stories all
illustrate this principle.

What is the best data will always change over time. Physicians
should adjust practice as it changes. If we acknowledge to our
patients and the public the uncertainty and the limits of the data
from the beginning, we need not react so drastically to new data.

On the other hand, if medicine continues to hide uncertainty
behind a face of determined confidence, we will continue to lose
face when our current practice is proven less than optimal by
future data. We cannot work so hard to convince the public that
we know everything and expect them simply to understand when
we have been dead wrong.

Dr. Goldstein says it never ceases to surprise him how difficult
it can be to communicate the omnipresent uncertainty to a jury.
When each jury member has likely seen many physicians, always
brimming with confidence, certitude, and rapid solutions for patient
complaints, of course they are surprised when the truth is told.

Starting Your Conversation. . . .

Oil Slick

Principle: Physician preferences dictate answers to many of the uncertainties among treatment options. Physicians vary as to how aggressive they are in erring on the side of over-treatment or under-treatment.

Ask your physician: What treatment do you prefer to provide for my condition? What treatment would you prefer to receive if you had my condition? Among specialists in your field, how many have the same preference? What is another common preference?

Principle and Interest

Principle: The mere perception that a treatment has been provided can powerfully affect patients, convincing them that receiving it improved their health.

Ask your physician: Has this treatment ever been compared head-to-head against a placebo?

Bucking

Principle: Financial conflicts of interest abound in medical treatment decisions. The most fundamental conflict of interest is that in many systems physicians are paid either to provide or withhold services.

Ask your physician: What do my different options cost? Who stands to gain or lose from the larger or smaller costs?

Mind the Gap

Principle: Most questions in medicine have not been studied carefully.

Ask your physician: Has my condition or this treatment been studied? What types of studies?

New Flash

Principle: Fads in medicine shift toward and away from certain treatments. Sometimes, the reaction to new evidence is stronger than really merited by the data, because physicians are so embarrassed that they were previously wrong.

Ask your physician: Are you treating my problem the same way you did a decade ago? If not, what was wrong with the old way? What do we know about the long-term results of the new way?

Guilt

Principle: Our desire to have an improvement to offer can cloud our assessment of progress in any field.

Ask your physician: Knowing that you and I both want my condition to improve, do you believe that this new treatment actually improves it? Why do you believe this?

Vigorous Precision

Principle: Some treatments have logical concerns attached. Rather than side effects, they are more expected-effects that just happen to be undesirable.

Ask your physician: Has this treatment ever been compared directly against the prior standard treatment? What was better about it? What was worse? From the way you think it will work in my body, for what bad effects should I watch?

The Upper Crust

Principle: Physicians don't like to discuss certain complications of certain treatments, because they are uncomfortable to face and may be subtle enough to be ignored with a little effort.

Ask your physician: What complication of this treatment do you least like to discuss?

The End Result

Principle: We have no good ways of measuring quality in physicians or medical care other than outcomes. No central repositories of information can measure these well, because of the many factors that jumble the results.

Ask your physician: Have you sent other patients to this particular specialist? Did they have good outcomes, by your assessment?

Where it Hurts

Principle: Convincing people that Medicine cannot control treatment outcomes is especially difficult because many have been led to believe it can.

Ask your physician: What aspect of my intended course of treatment is out of your control, but worries you most?

ERR CORRECTLY

Don't Pass GO

"It really doesn't hurt much," she answered my unspoken question. "As long as I don't move, I'm reasonably comfortable."

Catherine lay there, quite still. She somehow managed to appear relaxed, even serene. Having passed the last few hours in her hospital room without morphine, her mind had cleared remarkably for her 87 years. That shouldn't have surprised me. Until the day before this morning bedside visit, she had lived in her own home, after all. Widowed a decade earlier, she managed life independently.

She continued in my own silence, "Kevin, may I call you Kevin? I wouldn't normally call a doctor by his first name, but you remind me so much of my grandson. May I?"

"Of course. Please call me Kevin."

"Kevin, thank you for sitting and waiting with me. I know that you are very busy. I expect my children will arrive any moment for our discussion. They knew we planned for 9 o'clock. They are just a bit out of sorts with all of this."

All of this was that Catherine had fallen the day before after missing a step on the curb by her mailbox. The fall had broken her hip, bringing her to the hospital by ambulance.

"Let me run through my options one more time, before they

get here. They will be all a-fluster as they arrive, but I want to be sure to get this right," she continued. "Basically, your team can fix my broken hip or treat it without surgery."

"Correct," I agreed. "The surgery brings some immediate dangers, but lying in bed for a couple weeks until the pain settles down enough to sit up carries others."

She continued, "But if I do the non-operative treatment, my chances of regaining enough strength to walk well again and stay living in my home are very slim."

"I expect so," I had to admit.

"But you and Dr. Roberts think my heart has a high chance of failing during surgery."

"Yes. Your cardiologist thinks that your heart is barely pumping enough to get you through regular days. The stress of surgery will present a much bigger challenge."

After a thoughtful pause, she continued, "He thinks I should do it, though."

"Yes, he does. It's a little funny. Usually, as a surgeon, I am begging the cardiologist to let me take a patient to surgery, not the other way around."

"He's just worried what a week and half or two in bed will do to my already failing heart. I might never get up again."

"You might not," I affirmed. "On the other hand, you also might not wake up after surgery."

"I know, but I have not yet decided which is worse."

As her son and daughter arrived, I watched her closely. More commanding matriarch than crippled elderly woman, she greeted them almost sternly, "Dr. Jones is a busy resident. He has things he has to get to. The three of us can catch up after we finish our business with him."

"Well, she must be feeling well," her son noted, happily. "She is back to her usual self. I like this much better than the confusion she had in the ER last night from the morphine."

"Yes. I feel much clearer now. Let's hear what Dr. Jones has to tell us."

With a nod from Catherine, I began. "Thanks so much for hurrying in. Your mother wanted me to be here to answer any questions you had about her decision. I also wanted to be here to meet you and review options."

"So what's the story? What needs to happen?" her daughter started, before a quiet look from Catherine calmed her escalating anxiety.

"Basically, your mother's broken hip presents a big challenge because of her heart. We can fix the hip with surgery, but that will seriously risk her life. Or we can care for the break without surgery."

"Oh, that sounds like the best," Catherine's daughter said, almost relieved that surgery wasn't a must. "Let's do that."

Catherine stopped her daughter. "Let Dr. Jones finish. The non-operative treatment has its own problems."

"But Mom, your heart can't take a surgery. You're barely getting by day-to-day in that old house all by yourself."

Catherine answered with forced calm. "But I definitely give up the house and independent life, as well as possibly walking if I don't do the surgery."

"I don't want to overstate this," I said. "We *can* treat hip fractures without surgery, despite the fact that hardly anyone does that these days. The main challenge is that her heart is so weak already; the two weeks in bed before starting to get her up to a chair may hurt it even more."

"There is simply no get-out-of-jail-free card for me, is there?" Catherine paused. "Well, I think I've made up my mind."

"What would you like us to do?"

"I want surgery. I know that it may kill me, but I am okay with that. I cannot imagine going on with life in a way that isn't what life is to me now. I don't want to die slowly in some nursing home in a wheelchair. I would rather get up and walk with a fixed hip or die trying."

I answered a few more questions from her children, then gave them time to discuss it alone. Catherine didn't change her mind. She knew the risks she took. She preferred them to the risks of trying to manage her broken hip in bed.

I booked the surgery for that afternoon.

She rolled smoothly into the operating room. As Catherine drifted off to sleep under the anaesthesiologist's medication, she maintained the same quiet composure she had had during our interview a few hours earlier. We positioned her on the padded OR bed. We could all hear her heart beat on the monitors. I painted her bared thigh with the dark soap, then stepped out to wash my own hands.

My professor was already at the sink in the hallway, scrubbing his hands and forearms. "Kevin, I talked again with her and her family later this afternoon. You're right. They're game for this. They know her chances are not good."

"They aren't good," I agreed. "Her heart may not be up to this."

"Well, we'll see soon enough." He kicked his waterspout off with his knee and backed into the operating room. I finished scrubbing, rinsed and followed.

We hung the drapes, in this case a clear shower curtain-like covering that sticks to the skin in the area for her surgery, sealing it off.

"Everybody ready?" I called out, mostly to the anaesthesiologist.

"Yup. Go ahead."

I pressed the blade to the plastic sheet stuck on the skin where my professor had marked a line.

"Don't dally on this one," he suggested.

I didn't need to be told twice. I quickly drew the scalpel along the plastic-covered flesh. He and I each grabbed a hook to pull the skin edges apart.

"I would just go straight down to bone on her."

I did, with another slash of the blade through the deeper tissues. We each placed deeper hooks to hold the muscle and skin back from the bone. So far, so good. I could still hear the slow but steady beep of Catherine's heart, keeping about halftime with my own.

"Drill with guide-pin, please."

The scrub nurse handed me a power drill with a metal pin attached, ready to pierce Catherine's bone. I passed the pin through the bone, across the break, and up toward her hip. Still beeping. Maybe this would work, after all.

For the next step, I passed a large bore drill bit over the pin to core out a hole through the bone for a screw to follow. As I pulled the drill from the new hole it had created, I heard what I had nearly begun to hope I wouldn't. Silence. That precious beep had stopped altogether.

Then commotion broke the serenity Catherine had commanded so carefully in her hospital room. The door banged open as a second anaesthesiologist wheeled a crash cart into the operating room. The nurse left her instruments and pulled back part of the drape to begin chest compressions from the far side of the OR bed. The first anaesthesiologist was pushing drug syringes into the IV. The second grabbed the defibrillator from his cart. My professor and I did the only thing we could at the moment. I grabbed the large screw from the instrument table and twisted it into her bone as fast as I could. My professor slapped a metal plate over that. We stepped back to allow the first shock from the defibrillator.

No beep returned. With the drill, I placed a smaller screw below the first. Another defibrillator shock. Still, no heart beat. My professor was already stapling the skin edges together before I finished a third screw. Another shock. He finished the staples. We spread another plastic sticky sheet over the loosely closed wound and pulled our other drapes out of the way of the CPR team.

After a few more minutes, and a few more shocks, the first anaesthesiologist admitted defeat. It was futile to fight longer for a heart that had shown no semblance of a response to anything we threw at it.

Catherine's decision was final.

Except for emergently evolving situations, we can always reconsider diagnosis. We can go back. We can even start over. Once we move from a diagnosis or even a working diagnosis to a treatment decision, we take action. We cannot undo action. Treatment action may not always lead to a state as stubbornly irreversible as Catherine's, but it can never be taken back entirely.

On Purpose

"You will always err," Dr. Johnston flatly explained to a small cluster of eager young surgical trainees, gathered around a radiology light board to ask his opinion on an upcoming case. "Joint replacement surgery is really just about knowing in which direction to err."

Richard C. Johnston's wisdom didn't come cheaply. As the youngest founding member of the Hip Society in 1968, he was the pioneer of hip replacement in Iowa.[1] After visiting Wrightington Hospital and the inventor of the total hip replacement, Sir John Charnley, Johnston returned to bring what he learned in England to the Midwest region of the United States. He later saw and participated in the development of knee replacement for arthritis as well. Across his career he performed more than 8,000 knee and hip replacements. He practiced through major technological changes in the implants themselves.

Stories about the operating room of his earlier surgical career describe anything but an abandonment of control to the whims of error. He asked visitors to his OR to watch silently. They were reminded tersely --- if not gruffly --- when they forgot this admonition. He operated with the same assistants every time. Together they developed a silent but practically humming rhythm. The assistants passed him instruments without even spoken requests. Execution of each step was determined and precise. Only during closure of the skin would Dr. Johnston break the silence with conversation or the telling of jokes.

I would err if I called his operating room an intensely high-pressured environment. No. It was simply a well-oiled machine. Everyone knew what to do, how and when to do it. Even his choice of implants demonstrated a determination on precision. As new implant technologies became available, he would change his program only incrementally. Dr. Johnston made sure to do enough cases in series after each change to permit tracking and evaluation of the new technology's results. Younger surgeons have built research careers from follow-up studies of his well-documented, regimented case series. Johnston's team's results were unassailable. Even some of the most recently updated technologies for implants have not improved appreciably upon his results with the earliest, simplest implants procured directly from Charnley's factory.

As much as Dr. Johnston strove for precision then in his clinical practice, he strives for precision in his communication to these trainees now. He considers it base foolishness to presume that one can achieve perfect execution of a surgery to fit prefabricated implants, available in only a finite number of sizes and shapes, to the ends of human bones that vary even side to side, let alone patient to patient.

"You will err," he reiterates. "Just make sure you err in the right direction."

Johnston's principle of erring on purpose applies more generally than joint replacement. Physicians manage some uncertainties of treatment by erring on the side of caution or erring on the side of doing more instead of doing less. They don't erase the uncertainty, but choose which type of uncertainty they prefer to avoid and which they prefer to experience.

Confounded

When Dr. Johnston started doing total hip and later total knee replacements, the "directions in which to err" were not yet defined. Such answers don't come quickly. The effects of decisions made in a moment in the operating room on the thirty-year result of a given type of surgery, take thirty years to sort out, at least. Of course, that is only if you keep track. Dr. Johnston retired from surgical practice in his sixties only to begin a new career in outcomes-database management. He manages a clinic program that collects quality of life measurements and questionnaires from every patient seen by the surgeons of the Department of Orthopaedics and Rehabilitation at the University of Iowa.

"If we're not collecting the information now, we will not be able to look back on it when we have a question in the future," he frequently tells his colleagues. The department has basically acquiesced to the culture of clinical quality-of-life measurement before, during and after treatment. Some physicians still grumble when they must wait for a patient to fill out forms on a computer, but mostly, they get it.

"In joint replacement," Johnston asserts, "more has been learned from large national registries than from more tightly controlled scientific clinical trials. If we collect detailed data on how patients are functioning before surgery, details about the surgery itself, and then details about its outcomes over time, we should eventually be able to tell which details matter," says Johnston. "The questions we can ultimately ask by looking back at registries entirely depend on the data we collect along the way."

The problem? Variability not related to the disease in question that nonetheless impacts function. Johnston cites an intriguing example: whether or not a patient graduated from high school or avoided cigarette smoking will impact knee function scores as much as a wildly successful total knee replacement. These so-called confounding factors seriously challenge the interpretation of any results. Accidental or intentional differences in some confounding factor between comparison groups can powerfully skew the results in one direction or the other. What if all the smokers end up in one particular group? While one might think that simply accounting for these unrelated group differences would render the data meaningful, such accounting isn't easily performed.

"We have no good measure of co-morbidities," Johnston complains. Co-morbidities are the unrelated medical problems that patients bring along with them whenever undertaking a surgery. "Let alone adverse life circumstances such as poor socioeconomic status, use of cigarettes, or simply a pessimistic view on life."

He continued, "We know people have unrelated challenges; we know beyond a doubt that these confounding factors affect a patient's function and the change in function that results from any surgery. Unfortunately, we have no clear adjustment factor or calculation to account for any of these effects."

Such confounding factors challenge the interpretation of data from any biological system, but can powerfully impact medicine. Humans have the capacity to make choices, including choices that impact their health and well-being for better or worse. Unfortunately, in the setting of outcomes database research, we know that confounding factors will lead us to err, but we know neither in which direction nor how far they will lead us astray.

Show and Tell

As the dermatologist approached my wife's ear with the circular blade intended to punch out a biopsy of a worrisome mole, I winced.

The twinge of pain she might feel didn't trouble me in the slightest. I winced because the physician wasn't wearing sterile gloves. Rather, he wore the blue kind out of the box on the wall. He hadn't prepared her skin with any soap. He had just swabbed it with an alcohol wipe.

I had to remind myself for the moment that I was Kevin, supportive husband to Arden, not Dr. Jones. She wasn't my patient. I trusted this physician immensely. I remembered that he did such biopsies many times every day of every work-week. They must generally turn out well, or he would have noticed, right?

Did I know that the many differences between my own biopsy methods and the way this excellent physician proceeded had any importance? My background training differed dramatically from his. I had learned sterile technique in an OR, implanting metallic devices into bones, probably the most frightening setting for infection in all of medicine. Was my translation of those OR principles to the execution of my clinic biopsies just overkill? I didn't *know* that my obsessive sterile technique mattered in the clinic.

I didn't know because, to the best of my knowledge, the question had never been studied.

Physicians only know the answers to questions that have been studied. Many questions have not been. Further, not all studies provide the same level of knowing. I love it when radio advertisements selling the latest ultra-prostate-vitamin or the next elixir of youthful skin claim that "studies show" this or that. Although the studies these commercials cite rarely do, the best studies will *show* rather than *tell* me the value of some drug or surgical procedure. How well they show depends on many factors.

The first value assessment is the scientific rigor of the study design. The second source of value is the applicability of the study's information to the patient in front of me. As studies hope to guide decisions, they will attempt to peg different results between two groups of patients to a specific decision made for patients in each group. Scientific rigor requires then that the only input difference between the groups is the decision in question. All other conditions are controlled, or the same between the two groups. Such experiments are very difficult --- if not prohibitively difficult --- to perform for medically related decisions.

Consider, for example, the decision to breastfeed or bottle-feed a newborn. Many studies have tried to compare these two methods of infant nutrition. No group of mothers I have ever met would let some study randomly assign them to breastfeed or not. Infant nutrition stirs too many emotions. So every study medicine performs to compare breastfeeding to bottle-feeding must assume that the mothers who choose one or the other don't differ by any other factor that might affect whatever outcome the study measures. Such an assumption is dangerous scientifically. Not only emotions but fashionable trends, educational background, work responsibilities, socioeconomic status and many other factors can affect the mother's decision. Many of these factors might also influence the outcome in question, be it intelligence testing or infection rates.

How well a study scientifically balances or removes confounding factors determines the value of the information it provides. Not every question is as difficult to study as the decision to breastfeed, but no question in medicine is easily studied.

This book has already discussed a number of randomized controlled trials, the most complex and scientifically robust form of medical experiment. These experiments enroll patients defined by a given diagnosis or medical situation, then randomly assign them to one treatment or another. But randomization by itself can only insure a balance of confounding factors if the groups are enormous in size. Another way to increase scientific rigor with smaller group sizes is to define strict, narrow study-entry criteria to keep patients with some major confounding factor out of both groups. This instead threatens applicability.

If we know that smoking has a dramatic effect on some outcome, we can either enroll enough patients to insure a close to equal number of smokers in each group by the random assignment, or we can exclude smokers from the study. Excluding smokers will permit smaller groups, because the outcomes will have a narrower range. The problem we create by excluding smokers from the study is that our study results will not then be applicable to any decisions physicians may face with patients who smoke.

A study's applicability depends on whether physicians can fit the real patients in front of them into the study's entry criteria. A study of lip balm in Eskimos living in Canada's Northern Territory cannot safely advise selection of lip balm for urban dwellers in Ghana.

We have not had yet, nor are we likely to have any time soon, sufficient energy and resources to subject every possible patient situation and every possible solution to it to a randomized controlled clinical trial. Not even close. Forget mention of the ever-increasing numbers of drugs, interventions, and technologies yet to be basically tested, let alone compared to existing standard options. In the meantime, we must make do with the information we have from the studies that have been performed. That said, we must also carefully acknowledge what they can and cannot tell us.

a.k.a.

Many studies cannot even directly address the questions for which we most need answers. The result that clinically counts from a given treatment may be too far delayed or too infrequent to be efficiently studied in an experiment. Hardly any trial can afford to wait for the twenty-five-year result of an intervention, even if that is the result by which we hope to judge the intervention.

When we cannot measure what matters, we measure instead what is measurable, and hope that it matters.

Just under half of one percent of patients undergoing total hip replacement will die from a pulmonary embolism. A pulmonary embolism is a blood clot that forms deep in the limb then dislodges, floating back to the heart and landing in a clogging position in the lung.

Although rare, these deaths are devastating complications. Most physicians and patients consider the rate of one out of two hundred patients dying in such a way far too high.[2] Death by pulmonary embolism is quite worthy of prevention, if prevention is possible. Everyone agrees on that. The way forward, of course, is far less clear.

Several classes of drugs thin the blood and can prevent clot formation. Each of these blood thinners has undesirable side effects as well, primarily bleeding. The route to a solution seems obvious. Simply randomize patients getting total hip replacement to either placebo or one of these blood thinners. Then measure the rates of death from pulmonary embolism in each group. To be fair on the flip side, also measure the incidence of major bleeding in each group.

Such a study has never been performed. It isn't that we have performed *no* study, just not *that* study. The number of patients required in each group to detect a difference in death by pulmonary embolism that at worst may be 0.5 percent is untenable.

In the absence of the ability to measure what matters, we fall all over ourselves to measure instead what is measurable.

Using very sensitive imaging for detection, we can identify subtle clots very commonly after hip surgeries. The vast majority of these detectable clots will never cause death by pulmonary embolism. Most will generate no meaningful symptoms whatsoever for the patient. The frequency of these image-detected-only clots is high enough to render differences *measurable* between groups of hundreds of patients instead of hundreds of thousands. Measuring the variable rates of these image-detected clots becomes a surrogate --- or replacement --- for the outcome that really matters.

The sticking point with surrogates doesn't come with scientific value. If we measure the rate of image-detected clots to be significantly lower among hip surgery patients receiving drug A compared to hip surgery patients receiving drug B, we can safely conclude that drug A performs better than drug B at *preventing image-detected clots* after hip surgery. We can't really conclude, as too often happens, that drug A performs better than drug B at preventing death by pulmonary embolism. The study never measured death by pulmonary embolism. We have difficulty knowing how well the incidence of image-detected clots relates to death by pulmonary embolism. It *is* much more measurable.

Surrogates may stretch our resources to provide excellent

experiments, but we should very warily apply results from those experiments to real patients with distinct, real outcomes in mind.

Puffing

A few interventions for a few disease states have been informed by sound experiments that measure outcomes that matter, rather than surrogates, and relate to a real population that real physicians encounter in practice. Physicians consider the value of these interventions to be "known." These standards of care are evidence-based. These truths cause the chests of most modern physicians to puff with confidence.

One can take these therapies to the bank. However, let us consider how we really know the best of these truths, before we all pull out our checkbooks.

I recall learning in medical school that aspirin is an evidence-based, death-preventing drug when administered following a heart attack. This certainly meant that one would be crazy not to employ such a measure if faced with a patient scenario that fit the criteria. It certainly meant that medical school professors would teach such interventions to medical students and residents as essentially fact-based. It didn't mean that aspirin always improved a patient's condition in the setting of a heart attack.

Remember, biological systems of any type are prone to variation, often distributed across a bell-curve. Responses to medical evaluations and interventions vary similarly. Physicians "know" the value of interventions that fall in the favorable side of the bell-curve more often than not. With regard to aspirin preventing deaths if given shortly after heart attacks, we mean that statistically more patients given aspirin will survive than those denied it.

The first few trials evaluating the use of aspirin following a heart attack actually identified no statistically significant difference.[3] Medical scientists didn't give up because our statistics are designed to find or not find a difference between two groups; statistics are rather lousy at confirming that two groups are really the same. Researchers might have been sure with each study that they hadn't yet proven that aspirin was better, but they were less sure that they had proven that it was the same as the placebo treatment.

The landmark study that ultimately established the value of giving aspirin after a heart attack proved it with confidence of 99,999 out of 100,000. The study included 8600 patients in each group. We therefore estimate that a random sampling of two 8600-patient groups from a single population could erroneously find the same survival difference between the groups by accident only 1 out of 100,000 attempts. Such numbers grant very strong physician confidence that the difference between the death rates in the two groups was real, not accidental. Physicians believe that aspirin saves lives when given after heart attacks. This is great news, right?

Patients' confidence comes as they feel better. Will my taking this aspirin prevent my own death? Well, maybe.

These statistics were not measuring how much aspirin helped or how many it helped. The statistics could only tell us that the groups receiving or not receiving aspirin were different in death rate. The effect size, what really matters to most patients, is completely distinct. In the 8600 people studied in each group, 188 more survived in the aspirin group than in the control group. Therefore, only 2 percent more of the patients taking the aspirin actually survived, not 99,999 out of a hundred thousand. Aspirin even hurt a few patients, doubtless. As disheartening as this is, remember that this is about as good as it gets in terms of medical knowledge. They measured an outcome that matters and found a confident difference, even if it is a difference that inspires little confidence.

You can plainly see the challenge of applying population-based principles to individuals. Where an individual falls on the bell-curve distribution of responses to the intervention in question will make all the difference in the world. Physicians will feel quite well acquitted of their responsibilities when they provide a treatment within a standard of care bolstered by evidence as strong as we have for aspirin. While certainly defensible and far from error, the treatment may then help, hurt or have absolutely no impact on the patient's symptom.

I don't suggest that physicians stop using population-based data to make individual recommendations to patients. I know of no better way to establish principles to guide these decisions. Nevertheless, uncertainty roars in the details. I fear that most patients don't appreciate what such population-based data really mean to them on an individual basis. An individual who experiences a good or bad outcome of treatment that his physician expects in one percent of patients still experiences one hundred percent of it. We can only measure probabilities in populations, not possibilities for one patient.

When privately discussing a patient we had evaluated and judged to have a fifty-fifty chance of success with a treatment we were about to begin, one of my trainees considered, "If I am this guy, I am hoping that the other guy that I am paired to out there is doing very poorly right now."

We both gravely smiled. It simply doesn't work that way. When facing medical uncertainty for myself, my loved ones or my patients, I don't face it as a population.

Chameleon

Along an obscure hallway on an upper floor of one of the many amalgamated buildings that comprise Johns Hopkins Hospital, there are two adjacent doors. On one, locked and never opened or even open-able, hang cartoons clipped from newspapers and magazines; they cover the door from lintel to floor and handle to hinge. I'm not sure, but their curator behind the door may occasionally replace one of the comics with a fresh offering. From their yellowing tatters, most declare that they have maintained their enshrined prominence for decades. Behind the cartooned door lie stacks of files and books that literally pile floor to ceiling and cover all of the small office. In the only file-free flooring rests the footprint of a small desk and chair, plus just enough space for the room's other door to swing open and close. Despite his tucked-away office and the quiet and unassuming character of the physician who fills its desk chair, Brent Petty is legendary among the medical students who roam the halls beyond the cartooned door.

For more than 20 years, Dr. Petty has taught the practical sessions covering the reading of EKGs that highlight every medical student's rotation on Internal Medicine. Even a number of my other professors there had learned how to interpret EKGs at the feet of Brent Petty. Interestingly enough, Dr. Petty has no specialty training in cardiology. At certain points along the nine-week course that he repeats five times each year, he will say with a dry smile, "That is a question for the *real* heart doctors. Here we only cover the basics that every physician must know about EKGs."

Dr. Petty's demeanor is matter-of-fact to a remarkable degree. He deliberately regiments and disciplines his thinking. How could one not do so and still manage to enjoy teaching the same EKG course five times each year for 20 years? The small, out-of-the-way location of his office always made me wonder: Was he underappreciated by his department? Or, more likely, had he simply never wanted to change his location after settling there?

Since my medical school years, through serendipitous connections, I have met some of Dr. Petty's siblings, all of whom live in the western half of the United States, where he grew up. Some of them have mused, "We never really knew what happened to Brent. He moved to Baltimore for his residency in internal medicine and then simply never left, even when multiple opportunities for ostensibly more prominent positions have been available to him."

From the little I know of him, I can guess what his response would be, "Why change when you have a program that works?"

My interactions with Dr. Petty extended beyond the EKG course he taught during my internal medicine rotation of third year. He hosted --- whenever medical students were interested in attending --- a monthly journal club focused on treatment decision-making. During my years of participation, we typically had five to ten students show up each month. One student would have selected and distributed ahead of time an article for discussion. The only selection criteria for this article were that it was a study of some sort, not just a topical review, and that it involved some treatment intervention. It could be a drug trial, a surgical trial or even the testing of psychological behavioral therapy.

The process of the journal club followed a detailed presentation with discussion of the methods used by the investigators. We would pick apart the clinical science, identifying where the authors had taken the easy method rather than the most scientifically rigorous. Where had they used surrogates? Where had they measured the outcome that mattered? How applicable were the results to real patient situations? Each criticism of or praise for the methods used built toward a final question. Dr. Petty would always conclude the session with this: "From this study, will you change your practice?"

Appreciating the cognitive inertia of a man as intelligent and regimented as Brent Petty made this final ruling of each journal club especially intriguing. Would this man, who never seemed to throw away a comic strip he liked, or toss a file, or change his office, or move, or even teach a different course, change his clinical decision-making from a paper?

The answer wasn't always "No!" If the investigators had performed the study well, providing scientifically sound results that were applicable to real-life situations he would face as a physician, Dr. Petty *would* plan to change his practice.

Not all physicians are this open-minded. At least, most are not as regimented in their willingness to let carefully critiqued evidence change their practice whether or not it agrees with their own presumptions.

Stephen Katz directs the National Institute of Arthritis and Musculoskeletal and Skin Diseases (NIAMS), the NIH Institute charged with advancing research in the fields of dermatology (his own specialty), rheumatology, and orthopaedics. While giving a presentation to the American Orthopaedic Association about funding for orthopaedic research, he asked a very important question to the audience of surgeons: "Is there any evidence that NIH-funded research has changed the clinical practice of orthopaedic surgery?"[4] Dr. Katz may not have meant to, but his question touched a nerve.

Monies assigned to the completion of large, expensive surgical trials may well generate evidence for or against certain treatments, but will orthopaedic surgeons providing care to American patients then appropriately utilize the tested therapies more or less? I am embarrassed to admit it of my own specialty, but the answer is not a resounding "Yes!" The long and sordid tale of the field of orthopaedic surgery ignoring its own clinical trials can be found in many journal articles in the medical literature. The only trial results that I have seen widely adopted are those that uphold the general inclinations of most surgeons anyway.

A physician with whom I trained in residency compared an orthopaedic surgeon's use of evidence to a drunken man's use of a lamppost. He will lean upon it --- to be sure --- when it is conveniently positioned to support him, but from it, he will never seek illumination.

Some uncertainties in treatment remain due to the many questions physicians have not yet studied and many more that they have studied only poorly. Other uncertainties persist because physicians fail to use the information that the world of medicine has bothered to gather. Of course, we only strive to learn what we can from new information if we admit what we don't already know.

Painting by Number

Due to the many potential flaws we have discussed, evidence available from clinical research can rarely conclude that a given therapy is either ideal or hopelessly useless. Evidence from clinical research *can* guide the expectations that physicians assign to the options available. Even this application is indirect in most circumstances. Unless faced with a patient whose personal and medical circumstances fully meet the inclusion criteria of a large randomized clinical trial that included every option actually available now to the patient, then knowledge gained from the trial can be applied only indirectly.

It will not surprise you that we have found a way to study this as well. We call the study of indirect application of information from published trials and patient series "decision analysis." Essentially, decision analysis attempts to quantify the all-important qualitative values of given outcomes. After categorizing all possible outcomes into groups, decision analysis researchers will interview individuals from the public, asking them to assign values to each potential outcome group.

You can see immediately the primary threat to applicability

of decision analyses. Values of studied individuals may have no agreement with values of any given patient facing the actual decision. Further, value applied to a theoretical outcome never actually experienced by the evaluator may have no relationship to the experience itself.

One of the first decision analysis studies in the field of orthopaedic surgery provides an excellent example.[5] It was published by one of my own professors one month after I began my own specialty training in orthopaedic surgery. I therefore remember it well. I have to say *remember* it because I cannot admit that it informs much of my thinking about its specific topic now. It evaluated the utility of pinning (or fixing with a screw) both hips at the same time a surgeon undertakes pinning of one hip as treatment for slipped capital femoral epiphysis.

Slipped capital femoral epiphysis, or SCFE (pronounced "skiffee," and used much more frequently than the mouthful of words that comprise the technical name) is a progressive deformity of the upper femur. This capital femoral epiphysis is the ball from the ball-and-socket joint of the hip. The "slipped" part of the name derives from the fact that the head of the femur has slipped off from its normal position atop the neck of the femur.

One might compare a SCFE to a fracture or broken hip, only a SCFE more typically progresses over weeks and months rather than milliseconds. Most commonly, SCFE affects young people in the midst of their last growth spurt. The best understanding that we have mustered is that the growth plate, focused on its growth spurt, becomes structurally weak, permitting a sideways, sliding deformation. On a radiograph, a SCFE looks like a single-scoop of ice cream sliding backward off its cone.

A few health conditions specifically raise a child's risk of developing SCFE, such as obesity and thyroid problems. Many patients, however, have no specific risk factor associated. I should more correctly state that we *identify* no specific risk factor in many individuals who develop a SCFE. We know that many without an identified risk factor nonetheless must have some unknown risk factor, manifest by the fact that they will later develop a SCFE in the other hip. Many, but not all. This possibility and the challenges it presents to practice prompted the decision analysis.

If a surgeon catches a SCFE early in its progressive deformity and pins it in place, or passes a large screw across the slip before it deforms further, the child will have a fairly normal hip for life. When adolescents arrive in the orthopaedic surgeon's office late in the course with severe deformity or so late that the head has actually dislodged entirely from the neck of the femur, the chances of having permanent hip problems increase dramatically. One undertakes pinning at some costs, though. I don't mean financial costs --- I mean costs in the form of unwanted outcomes like infection or erosion of the joint cartilage. You can see the same rock-and-a-hard-place scenario developing with this decision that is present in so many decisions in medicine. One must weigh risks and benefits. There may not be a *correct* answer.

This decision analysis developed probabilities of experiencing the entire range of possible outcomes from never developing SCFE-like problems in the second hip after not pinning it, to successfully pinning it and avoiding problems, to pinning it unnecessarily and developing terrible complications. The investigators gathered data from the published literature to inform how frequently each outcome would likely occur. Study participants from the public then graded each outcome category, assigning values. Special statistical modeling and tests spat out the recommendation that for most SCFEs presenting to medical attention, the surgeon should proceed with pinning both the SCFE and the other normal hip. The risks and benefits, each weighted by participants that had experienced neither, favored preventative pinning of the normal hip, just in case.

So what? What do we do with a study that carefully renders numerical values for the perceptions of uncertainty? I don't know what all children's orthopaedic surgeons do across the country. I do know what the senior author on that paper happens to do: he almost never pins the other normal hip. Why? Does he consider his own paper invalid? No. Rather, he trusts his conversations with patients more than he trusts the theoretical assessments of value.

Perhaps choosing by numbers, in cases such as this, mirrors painting by numbers, fine for the amateur, but a little boxy and oversimplified to the trained eye.

I read recently that the Chevron Corporation won an award from the Decision Analysis Society because they guide all their business decisions by decision analysis. Critically, though, their decisions concern a substance derived from organic material that has rotted beneath the earth's surface for thousands of years, not the hip of a 12-year-old.

Humans, not computers, make medical decisions. Human interaction based entirely upon cut-and-dried algorithms would be frank insanity. Even that presumes that the numbers are indeed cut-and-dried. Regarding pinning both hips when one SCFE is diagnosed, another decision analysis study was published by some other experts in the field two years after the first. It advanced the opposite conclusion. Now each surgeon can pick which study to believe. She will have to err in one direction or the other. Ideally, she will err correctly.

Because adequately gathered numbers are lacking for most medical situations and are imperfectly applicable in all medical situations, I bristle a little at the recent popularity of treatment guidelines set by panels of experts. These have become the major means by which medical societies try to influence and control the standards of care for their respective specialties. They tend to derive from a thought process not unlike decision analysis, only less statistically rigorous. You can see from the two SCFE decision-analyses that even experts using the best information available and the most careful statistical methods can generate completely opposite recommendations. Managing uncertainty in treatments cannot help but be messy. Ignoring this fact can make it messier.

While you have heard me criticize my own specialty for ignoring some of the evidence available to it, I worry as much or more about the prospect of top-down standards imposed as guidelines, checklists and quality measures. Insofar as these can be based on sound evidence, they might be reasonable, but you have seen how sound (really unsound) most of our evidence is for treatment decisions in the world of medicine. What is the best evidence for a given situation? Who chooses what is best? What influences their decisions? Do they account for confounders? Do they use evidence from trials employing surrogates just because they are scientifically strong? Do they pay attention to the effect sizes of the trials whose data they want to apply?

Guidelines as a means of managing uncertainty in treatment can make that uncertainty seem much less real than it really is. I worry that standards imposed from above only discourage physicians from knowing and remembering how fuzzy the actual evidence is for many of the treatment decisions they face with their patients. Guidelines make an accepted standard treatment the apparently cut-and-dried answer for a given clinical situation but bring physicians no closer to the certainty of truth.

I favor, instead, honesty as the principal means of managing uncertainty in treatment. Let me be clear with a patient when we are guessing and how we are making that guess our best guess.

Starting Your Conversation. . . .

Don't Pass GO

Principle: Once we choose a diagnosis and act on it, we cannot usually start the process over.

Ask your physician: As we will never be at exactly this same point again, is there anything we should check before we start changing things with treatment?

On Purpose

Principle: Given that we essentially never get something exactly correct in biological systems, we must choose in which direction we will err.

Ask your physician: For my condition, are you aiming initially for over-treatment or under-treatment? Avoiding risks or maximizing benefits?

Confounded

Principle: Other matters of life and health dramatically affect how much of a problem any specific diagnosis will be for our well-being. This challenges the measuring of these effects as well, if comparison groups in a study have unrelated differences that affect outcome.

Ask your physician: Is there anything about my other health or life situation that worries you with regard to the impact of this upcoming treatment? Can I change any of those factors?

Show and Tell

Principle: We can only really know the answers to questions that have been very carefully tested in well-crafted scientific studies. Not all studies give us the same level of confidence in the answers they provide.

Ask your physician: Has this treatment ever been studied directly? Do you trust the design of the study?

a.k.a.

Principle: Rather than measuring the outcome that really matters, some studies measure surrogate outcomes that are more easily measured, hoping that the surrogates reflect the rates of the meaningful outcomes.

Ask your physician: In achieving or avoiding what outcome are you most interested with this treatment? Has anyone ever measured that specific outcome following this treatment?

Puffing

Principle: Even randomized controlled trials with statistically significant results may find such small effect sizes that the intervention promises very little overall to patients.

Ask your physician: What is the effect size of this intervention in the population treated? How many people in my situation will you have to treat before you will see one success?

Chameleon

Principle: Too few physicians allow new information from rigorously scientific studies to change their practice. Physicians willing to change, when the evidence is strong enough, may be those most determined to stick rigidly to principles, rather than to stick stubbornly to their own opinions.

Ask your physician: Have you read any study recently that changed your practice in this area?

Painting by Number

Principle: Because evidence is never perfectly prescriptive, we can apply it only indirectly to most situations. Researchers have studied the process of adding value-assessments to expected outcome scenarios.

Ask your physician: What is the range of outcomes I could expect from each option?

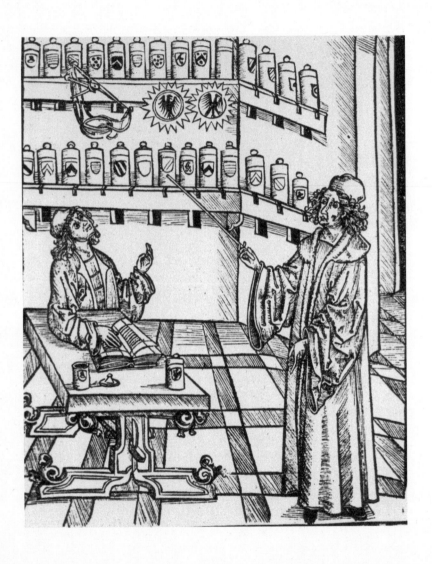

WHEN TO SAY "WHEN"

Picking Poison

Kate's cancer responded dramatically to her initial course of chemotherapy. It responded so dramatically that the pathologist found no living cancer cells in the tumor we removed from Kate's thigh, only residual scar tissue. This 100 percent tumor necrosis, or "complete" pathologic response to the chemotherapy given before surgery, told us that the selected chemotherapy regimen was working. It also indicated Kate's high chances of ultimately winning her fight against cancer. We discussed these delightful findings about two weeks after a major surgery to remove the tumor and rebuild her limb. More emotional than I had yet seen her, Kate shed bitter tears despite this good news.

"So I don't get to stop chemotherapy any earlier?" she asked, knowing what my answer would be.

I knew how difficult chemotherapy had been for Kate. No one enjoys the aggressive chemotherapy given for sarcomas, but some fare worse than others. Kate had especially struggled. Most experience some measure of hair loss, mouth sores, nausea, vomiting and general fatigue. Kate had taken these in stride. She had been more discouraged by the short-term memory loss that had plagued her during each dose of a particular drug called ifosfamide. For an extremely bright high school student, fluent in five languages and socially engaging, these weeklong mental lapses were horrifying.

The severity of the symptoms had sufficiently worried us that her chemotherapy doctor and I acquiesced to Kate's pleading to move her surgery up a couple of weeks in order to delay the next treatment with ifosfamide until after surgery. We wanted the tumor necrosis percentage from the pathologist to confirm that poisoning her brain with ifosfamide was at least also accomplishing something meaningful in terms of tumor kill.

No imaging or blood test can predictably measure the effects of the chemotherapy on tumors like Kate's. We depend on the pathologist's assessment of the removed tumor. This pathologist's inability to identify any living tumor cells in the bone where Kate's cancer had started confirmed a remarkable response to the chemotherapy. Indeed, the tumor had responded far better than we had guessed from the imaging, rendering this good news somewhat of a surprise.

"No," I responded in a metered word. "This gives us confidence that the chemotherapy regimen you have been receiving is working. This tells us that, as best we can project, even the bad chemo [her name for the ifosfamide] will probably be worth it in the end."

"So I have to keep getting the ifosfamide?"

"As you know, you don't *have* to do anything. My best advice to you would be to continue your chemotherapy regimen. You may now steel yourself with the knowledge that it is, by our best measure, working to kill your cancer."

Kate's father interjected: "We only want what is best. Kate can handle more ifosfamide if it is the best way to kill the rest of her tumor."

"But do I have any more tumor? You said you got it all out of my thigh with negative margins. You said that even the tumor that was there was completely dead. How do I still have tumor?"

"I hope you don't," I offered.

"What do you mean?" she asked.

"I hope that every treatment you receive from this point forward is overkill. I hope that you are already entirely free from that cancer."

"But…" Kate looked exasperated.

"But I don't *know* that you are tumor-free. Neither do I have any way of knowing that you are."

"What about my scans?" Kate was asking about the CT scan of her lungs and bone scan of her skeleton. These scans screen for any sites of metastatic disease from the cancer that originated in her femur.

"As you know, your scans are negative. However, scans are not perfect in their detection. The CT scan cannot identify lung spots smaller than three or four millimeters. The bone scan only detects spots about two or three times that size."

Now Kate's mother joined in. "How can we keep giving her these poisons if they might not be necessary? Why would we do that?"

"All we know is that in large groups of patients treated with these regimens, more of those with 100 percent necrosis, or optimal treatment effect, at surgical resection are alive at five years after surgery. All of them still received the post-operative chemotherapy. Not giving the post-operative chemotherapy hasn't been tried in a group of patients where preoperative chemotherapy worked this well."

"Why not?"

"The stakes are simply too high."

Ultimately, Kate and her parents did understand the uncertainty of her situation. They also understood that a choice to proceed was the best means of avoiding the worst result. They accepted this as our only rational answer to the uncertainty.

When a new treatment renders a previously non-survivable disease sixty percent survivable, one then chooses to scale back that treatment due to side effects only with great trepidation. The risk of losing that improved survival in exchange for less morbid treatment powerfully impedes trying anything less aggressive. The chance of a high-stakes failure often prevents incremental improvements in something that generally works.

This is difficult to explain to patients. People fail to recognize that every improvement begins as a change that may impact success in the wrong direction.

In another type of bone cancer, osteosarcoma, physicians didn't attempt the use of chemotherapy of any kind until the mid 1970s.[1] Prior to that time, surgeons treated the disease with amputation alone. Between 10 and 20 percent of patients treated with surgery alone survived in the long run. That rate of survival nearly turned upside down with the use of aggressive chemotherapy. Survival increased to around 70 percent. Medicine evaluates such a tripling to seven-fold multiplication of survival as a slam dunk of a success in terms of medical advances.

No one questions the utility of cytotoxic chemotherapy for osteosarcoma, but it isn't without its drawbacks. Following chemotherapy, we expect that around one percent of patients will eventually develop a second cancer. Others' hearts will fail because of difficulties from one of the drugs. A few will die from complications during the treatment itself. You would happily accept these tradeoffs if you're one of the 50 to 60 percent of those treated who survive but wouldn't have in the surgical-treatment-only days. If you're among the 10 to 20 per cent who would have survived without chemotherapy, having had surgery alone, you would find these side effects less emotionally tolerable. Of course, we cannot identify even in hindsight which of these two groups would have included any given survivor. That remains uncertain.

We will always either over-treat or under-treat every troublesome medical condition. To manage some incurable but chronic conditions we can slowly titrate our treatments to the desired effect, adjusting to more and less aggressive treatments as we go. Cancer is different. With cancer, our first shot is by far our best. Clinical progression of cancer frequently proves to be an irreversible event, beginning an inexorable course toward the patient's demise. For cancer, therefore, we always hope to over-treat the first time.

Avoidance of progression justifies incredible morbidity from the side effects of any treatment. Because we also don't like these morbid side effects, we hope to over-treat just slightly. Our fear of approaching that deadly under-treatment threshold prevents our titrating cancer treatments very tightly.

Marginal Circumstance

Jeff is about as athletic as a 45-year-old can be without being a professional athlete. As a U.S. Air Force reservist helicopter pilot, he has served multiple tours of duty, including a stint in Afghanistan. He splits his civilian time with a job as a commercial airline pilot, a hobby as a high-risk, high-altitude rescue-mission helicopter pilot, and a passion for ironman triathlons and the training they require. I use the present tense incorrectly. Before he came to see me, Jeff split his time this way.

Jeff came to see me because hip pain interrupted his last tour in Afghanistan. It began late in the course of his daily multiple-mile runs. The onset of a click in his hip ultimately punctuated this pain. This click bothered him enough to stop his runs altogether. As his tour finished, he saw his physician, who ordered some radiographs of the hip.

Something "a little funny" on his radiographs prompted further three-dimensional imaging.

Something downright alarming on the three-dimensional imaging prompted referral to my clinic.

A mass had destroyed the bone immediately adjacent to the supporting structures of the hip socket, or acetabulum. This mass easily explained his pain. It also explained the click in his hip: the tumor had grown into the hip joint itself in one place. The tumor's appearance bore characteristics of something called a chondrosarcoma. Part of this presumed-chondrosarcoma had eroded through the bone's surface to produce a continuous mass into the soft tissues.

"I want you to take my leg off," Jeff opened our conversation.

Surprised by his abrupt salutation, I was unable to speak.

Jeff plowed on.

"I want you to take my leg off. I have been reading a lot about this. I know that I will probably die anyway, but I want you to take my leg off. Sports are very important to me. I understand that I will be better able to participate in sports without a leg than with a lousy leg. I want you to take my leg off."

I reinitiated the conversation. "I am Kevin Jones. May I ask you a few questions before we jump to the conclusion of removing your limb?"

Jeff started in again with his very determined statement of

purpose. He had visible difficulty keeping at bay the emotions that were boiling beneath his planned stoicism.

"Mr. Stevens," I interrupted more forcefully, "let me quickly give you my assessment of your imaging findings, because it appears that you have drawn conclusions from them with which I may not fully agree. After I explain my first-pass impression from the imaging, maybe you can then tell me more about how you came to know about this in the first place and then more about what you have been told so far."

He took a step back, then sat rigidly in a clinic room chair. He listened as I explained briefly what I knew so far. The tumor in his pelvis wasn't likely to kill him. It was also compatible anatomically with limb-salvage, our technical word for tumor removal without amputation of the involved limb. He had what he could expect to be a body-and-life-changing operation ahead of him, but he would optimally complete that operation with his limb still attached and generally functional.

Jeff explained how he came to know of the mass in his pelvis bone, as well as what he had been told about it. A physical examination followed this interview. We reviewed the imaging studies in greater detail together. We then agreed on the next step: confirm or refute the diagnosis of chondrosarcoma that I suspected. Jeff would see a radiologist who would use guidance by CT scan to snake a large needle through the muscles in front of his hip to sample the bone and soft-tissue mass underneath. A pathologist would then render an opinion on the diagnosis from this small sample.

When the pathologist confirmed the diagnosis of chondrosarcoma, Jeff and I met again to discuss it. I came to learn that his original penchant for amputation was based on appreciation of the fact that many amputees are much more functionally athletic than they could be with metallic implants replacing parts of their bones. The type of amputation that could remove Jeff's tumor, however, wouldn't likely result in athletic participation. Prosthetic limbs provide very little function without a hip to support them. Jeff began to back away from the limb-removal option. His tough decisions were not yet over.

Due to the precise location of his tumor, I felt that we could safely remove the entire hip joint in a way that would permit reconstruction to support the limb below. He would have enough of the supporting bone left from the rear side of his pelvis that I could attach with screws the socket side of a total hip replacement. This should make him much more functional than limb removal or limb salvage with a flail hip would permit.

The only catch? Bone stability is only one of the issues. Soft-tissue function is another. The tumor's extension beyond the pelvis bone into the soft-tissues compromised one particular muscle group. Furthermore, the needle biopsy tract had pierced through the same muscles. The potentially contaminated muscle group normally powers hip flexion, the lifting of the thigh and knee in front of a person. I recommended removal of these muscles as a margin on the tumor. I also acknowledged that this recommendation was controversial and that I fell on the aggressive side of the spectrum of how much of a margin is enough. Specifically, sarcoma surgeons hotly debate whether or not they should treat needle tracts as if they are part of the cancer.

In a recent research meeting, one senior surgeon stood and proclaimed that a single-cell width beyond the tumor provides a sufficient margin. Most present at the meeting chuckled uncomfortably at this statement. Of course, everyone agreed that one cell width beyond the tumor is enough; but one cell width into the tumor isn't enough. We don't always know pre-operatively or even intra-operatively where, on a cellular level, that critical distinction between tumor and normal tissue lies.

I often explain to my patients that removing a sarcoma-type cancer is like removing a yolk from a hard-boiled egg. We want to open the skin or crack the shell, then dissect through the white to remove the yellow yolk without ever seeing it during the operation. We then hand what appears to be a white ball to the pathologist, who slices it in half to tell us how thick the layer of white really is around the yellow. That thickness is our margin.

Tumors don't usually have an egg's white/yellow, blatantly apparent border with the enveloping normal tissues. No one can readily discern the border to that level of detail on imaging studies such as the MRIs that we use to plan most sarcoma surgical resections.

Dissection of sarcoma surgical specimens has identified unmistakable tumor cells up to 5 cm beyond the apparent tumor border.

To complicate things further, every tumor is different. Each surrounding tissue type is unique as well. Tissues packed densely with tough collagen fibers contain tumors more tightly in narrow margins. Muscles are not such a tissue. Muscles don't predictably contain tumors within millimeters of the apparent yellow/white border. This variability explains the small but real rates of tumor recurrence following what were considered by a pathologist to be free, or negative, margins (a continuous white layer with no yellow peeking through). Ask surgeons how much is enough, and they will frequently disagree, both generally and given the unique circumstances of the given case.

Jeff understood that it was up to him to decide. I could ignore the needle tract and keep the thinnest margin possible against his tumor or, alternatively, remove his hip flexors as a wider margin.

What did the first option risk? A higher chance for leaving microscopic tumor cells behind, it slightly increased the risk for recurrence of the tumor.

What might that mean? Well, it is difficult to "win" in the pelvis at all and nearly impossible to win in a second surgery when the first one fails to eradicate a tumor. This might result in later loss of limb or even progression to metastatic disease and death. And what was at stake with the more surgically aggressive option, removing the muscles? Loss of hip flexion. While the chances of the worst-case scenario from leaving the muscles were very small, the chance of losing hip flexion power from removing the muscles was 100 percent.

As many do, Jeff asked for my opinion. I explained that I preferred to remove the muscles, with the caveat that I knew other surgeons who definitely would not. He decided to follow my preference. Perhaps he trusted me. Perhaps he is also very risk-averse personally. I find the explanation of his own risk aversion somewhat hard to imagine given his high-risk profession and hobbies.

Now far to the other side of that decision, Jeff's rehabilitation has returned him to a level of athleticism that I will never even hope to attain myself. But he has poor hip flexion power. I know that he doesn't look back pensively on that decision. I do look back on my advice to him. For most patients, I can safely ignore as negligible the functional implications of hip flexor resection, but for Jeff, they significantly impact his sports involvement.

The flavor and feeling of the discussions regarding the removal of those muscles would be different with every surgeon with whom he could have had them. This fact should not, perhaps, but does astonish me. I doubt many surgeons would even bother to discuss it, no matter which side of the decision they preferred. The choice would usually be the surgeon's alone. Perhaps it should be. Did I truly apprise Jeff of all the information in sufficient detail that he could make a decision independent of my preference?

I believe that a patient deserves to understand the surgeon's self-assessment of his general flavor and feelings. Does the surgeon tend to make gray into black or white? Does he do his very best to avoid danger for or to maximize gain for patients?

While a patient may see either one of us when referred with a sarcoma, my partner and I don't entirely agree on such judgments for individual cases. Each of us puts his very best effort into such judgments, but the feel and flavor differ. My colleague strives to see how much muscle he can get away with saving without detrimentally affecting local recurrence. I strive to see how wide a margin I can maintain on the tumor without detrimentally affecting function. Often these flavors align our judgments precisely, even if we arrived from different directions. Not always.

Which is right? I have no idea, but each of us is aware that he has an approach. I think we both agree that patients deserve to know our basic approach. The real question becomes, is one approach better than the other?

Sidestep

I choose to discuss uncertainty with my patients because I believe it is the most honest and humble path forward, but acknowledging uncertainty functions beyond this sense of integrity. Acknowledgement takes the first step toward reducing uncertainty in the future. I am not intentionally hearkening to the philosophy behind the Alcoholics Anonymous steps, but it may also apply. More directly, if we cannot acknowledge uncertainty between two available treatment approaches, how can we convince ourselves to enroll patients into randomized controlled trials actually comparing the two?

We can't study every question most practically with a randomized controlled trial, but a randomized controlled trial provides the only method of study with any chance of meaningfully distinguishing two relatively similar treatments. No other method controls for as many confounders and sources of bias.

Prior to enrollment in a trial, the patient has come to see a physician seeking a solution for some symptom. That physician has made a diagnosis and prepared to offer therapy. Then the physician must explain that there are two options and that he has no idea which one is better. Both have risks. Both have potential benefits. The physician doesn't know which is better overall.

This balancing concept is called "equipoise." A physician with equipoise feels that two options are equivalent and presents them as such. This conversation can go well as long as the physician actually has no opinion about which option is better. Rarely do physicians honestly lack such opinions.

"You have to take the physician out of it," says James N. Weinstein, the recent principal investigator on one of the largest orthopaedic surgical trials ever undertaken.[2] For this trial, his team developed an elaborate nurse-administered video instruction session for each patient to experience after a physician judged that the patient met study entry criteria. "Our enrollment in the randomization arm went way up with this system," Dr. Weinstein explains.

Nonetheless, their enrollment lagged behind that for drug trials. That his physicians were necessarily surgeons partly challenged Dr. Weinstein's trial enrollment. For patients and their surgeons, decision-making differs dramatically from that between patients and physicians offering drug therapies. As in all medical treatment encounters, a patient wants a surgeon to provide a solution to his symptom, a fix for his problem. Unique to surgery, however, the surgeon *is* the solution.

Rather than merely directing one toward it, surgeons personally enact or perform the solutions they offer. You may take an orange pill from any variety of physicians, but the hip surgery or bladder surgery or neck surgery performed by one surgeon, rather than another, may not be as standard as the orange pill. You want your surgeon to be good. You may not care one bit for his bedside manner. You want him to cut and sew well, with skill and precision.

Worst of all, you have no way of assessing surgeon quality. Instead, you base your judgment on a variety of likely meaningless clues. When considering a surgery, patients have the perception, correct or incorrect, that confident decision-making in the clinic may translate into confident (and hopefully correct) decision-making in the operating room. Busy surgeons know how to score confidence points with patients.

The very nature of surgery itself attracts medical students with more confident personalities to surgical specialties for residency. It is often quipped that surgeons are "sometimes in error, but never in doubt." Functionally, especially during surgery, surgeons must fill in gaps in knowable certainty with decisive, sometimes bold action. Those attracted to this type of decision-making comprise a rather bullish subgroup of physicians.

My father, also a surgeon, still laughs at a comment I made to him during my first year in medical school. I said, "Dad, there is a very fine line between frank hubris and the confidence it takes to think it is a good idea to cut someone open and rearrange anatomy."

"I never really thought of it that way," he had responded. "That is probably why you will never be a surgeon."

My father, actually a very thoughtful man, may have never questioned the value of cutting someone open and rearranging anatomy when it was anatomically awry. His point in doubting at that moment that I would end up pursuing a career in surgery was simple. It takes such an incredible dose of confidence to perform the violence that surgery is on the human body that few can manage to do it reflectively.

There is no place in the operating room for a Hamlet, mired in reflective indecision. The operating room is a place of action. It is a place where surgeons must transform gray expeditiously into either black or white.

This confidence challenges decision-making outside of the operating room, especially the decision to randomize a patient in a surgical trial. To enroll a patient in a randomized trial, the surgeon has to reflect for a moment of equipoise. The surgeon must cast doubt on whether his efforts in the operating room will actually accomplish anything positive for the patient, compared to choosing a nonsurgical option.

Reflecting on that doubt, no matter how omnipresent it may be in surgery, is rather uncomfortable for surgeons, even in private. It is downright excruciating for most surgeons to cast doubt on surgery in front of a patient. "Maybe the patient will think that surgical success is only doubted when I perform the surgery," some will reason. "I know he can go across town to Dr. So-and-So who will tell him that her surgery works every time."

Medicine generally --- and surgery especially --- subjects patients to invasive and uncomfortable treatments. These treatments are also uncertain in both the benefits they offer and the risks to which they expose patients. Pursuing these uncertain treatments requires gumption. This confidence can spill over easily into arrogance. Most would agree that arrogance is an annoying character trait, but it is also dangerous when it drives decision-making.

The classical Greek tragedy, *Oedipus Rex*, teaches about the danger of arrogance in decision-making. Blinded by arrogance, Oedipus kills his father and marries his mother, the exact choices he planned to avoid. As the play ends, he gouges out his eyes as he realizes just how blind he has been. So, confidence-enabling decisions is necessary and good, but arrogance can dangerously blind us. Unfortunately, in the muddle of medicine and surgery one must ask how many physicians depend on a little blindness for their basic confidence in the first place?

As patients and physicians can we tolerate honesty? Can we still muster the gumption necessary to undertake what may be brutal treatments even after acknowledging the uncertainties involved? I believe we can. Not everyone will agree.

Dosing Nonsense

The emotional and psychological impacts of uncertainty on communication regarding treatment are neither new, nor newly recognized. In 1672, a French physician, Samuel de Sorbiere, wrote a book entitled *Advice to a young Physician Respecting the Way in Which He is to Conduct Himself in the Practice of Medicine.*[3] De Sorbiere satirized the prospect of a physician disclosing the imperfect science of medicine to a patient. He considered it laughable.

He advised his audience of young physicians to keep handy a "few doses of nonsense to bestow" upon patients with questions. The necessity de Sorbiere saw for dishonesty was patient retention. He admonished that when faced with full acknowledgment of uncertainty in a physician, patients would naturally seek another physician. These days, no one claims such thinking quite as boldly as de Sorbiere. But that sentiment remains entrenched in the practice of medicine, especially surgical specialties.

A patient of mine recently transferred her care to me against the will of her local surgeon. She drove herself three hours and checked in to our University Hospital emergency room. She told me that she had requested a second opinion at our center for the evaluation of her thigh mass, but was discouraged from this. The local surgeon felt that she might not have cancer. He had explained that he would be embarrassed to consult our team if her mass ended up being benign.

I may not fully appreciate his thoughts, receiving them third-hand through my patient. I fear that they display the same thinking de Sorbiere expressed. This surgeon feared more the loss of the patient than potential embarrassment. Why would he say this to a patient --- as an assertion of confidence? I have never and would never chastise any referring physician for referring a patient before cancer was confirmed. Did he really think I would?

I understand the local surgeon's sentiment. He can't enjoy losing a patient because she doesn't trust his ability to handle her surgical condition. Establishing trust with patients is difficult. Still, must we resort to lies to achieve it? I personally try to avoid de Sorbiere's "nonsense."

Nonetheless, I often find myself trying to reassure patients that the doubts I feel obligated to cast on certain surgeries are not doubts in my capacity to perform them well. I strive to distinguish that my doubts are doubts in the value of the interventions themselves. As I have not observed patients fleeing my office in droves, most apparently believe me. It can be a difficult distinction, though. Inspiring confidence in the presence of acknowledged doubt is very difficult for surgeons.

I hope that answers other than simply removing surgeons from pre-operative decision-making and trial enrollment present themselves. Many medical systems employ such divisions of labor. In German health care, most surgical subspecialties have surgical and non-surgical practitioners. The former counterparts spend their time almost exclusively doing surgery in hospitals. The latter staff clinics and decide which patients should be scheduled for which surgery. The surgical surgeons become more like a pharmaceutical company, providing the orange pill.

In the United States, some surgical specialties approach this model. Medical endocrinologists often refer patients to thyroid and parathyroid surgeons; such patients are essentially ready for and already determined in favor of surgery. Cardiac bypass specialists usually work closely with cardiologists, who have significant discretion on whom to refer for bypass surgery.

Surgeons *should* guide their patients through surgical decisions. If only we can suppress our own insecurities and find confidence more in honesty than bravado, we might begin to provide this critical service.

Intrepid

It all comes down to confidence. It seems that the more uncertain a treatment decision is, the more confidence patients expect from their physicians. I have specifically decried surgeons' ability to recruit patients to clinical trials. That may not be entirely fair. I wish that surgeons would redirect some of their confidence away from their prowess in the operating room and toward their ability to counsel well with patients, but they are not the only ones that struggle in recruiting patients to randomized trials.

Even among non-surgical specialties, recruitment to randomized trials is very difficult. Some develop honed skills in recruitment. Many academic physicians make a career of this skill. Intriguing to me, one of the best recruiters to clinical trials in my state of Utah is, interestingly enough, a non-academic physician. Personally, he stands to gain little from his trial recruitments. Nathan Rich works in a solo medical oncology practice in a smaller outlying town. In this unlikely setting, he recruits more patients to clinical trials than most of the medical oncologists at our large university center. He recruits more than any of those associated with the other large private tertiary medical center in our state.

Dr. Rich doesn't consider himself a great clinical scientist. He serves as the principal investigator, or study initiator, of none of the trials to which he recruits patients. None of the publications that will result will likely list his name. He has no financial relationships with any drug companies whose drugs the trials test.

If Nathan learns of a patient's eligibility for a trial at our university cancer center that isn't available through his practice, he will refer the patient to see the appropriate oncologist at our center. He will go so far as to take pains to facilitate their care with his theoretical competitor.

We may never comprehend his motivation.

I worry little about Dr. Rich's *why*; let us try to understand his *how*.

Out of training only five years, Nathan Rich considers himself relatively young and relatively new to his current practice situation. Nevertheless, medical uncertainty doesn't frighten him.

He employs a very simple method to encourage enrollment in clinical trials: honesty. Nathan points out to his patients what benefits of knowledge gained from prior trials they personally reap. He also reminds patients of those following them, their own children or grandchildren possibly included, who will benefit from what the ongoing trials can teach us. "Let us do what we know every time. When we pass what we know, let us be guided by enrollment in a trial protocol to force the gray void into black and white, rather than some random singular opinion. There isn't a trial available for every situation and circumstance, but when there is one. . . ."

Nathan's demeanor, or "bedside manner," as we often name physician interpersonal skills, disarms with a quiet confidence. He knows that he doesn't know everything. He cannot control everything. Those facts don't fluster him one bit.

It almost seems that he lets his patients borrow his own courage, whether they are facing enrollment in a trial or choosing hospice and supportive care only rather than aggressive uncomfortable treatments with little foreseeable benefit. He is a gifted communicator. He communicates not as a politician or salesman, slick at the job of convincing you of his way. Nathan inspires patients to make decisions bravely and honestly, rather than from fear of the unknown alone. He communicates as an educator, not a solicitor.

This may be every physician's primary job. It is a difficult job. It is also a job for which no physician receives any real training. I am not certain how the rest of us can learn to communicate as well as Nathan does. We invest great effort in learning the opposite.

Much of medical education and training impedes the trainee's ultimate role as an educator to the lay public on a one-by-one basis. We spend our education learning the language, lingo, and jargon of medicine, "Doctorspeak," if you will. We learn the Latin and Greek names of anatomic parts, despite the fact that most of those names are only descriptive in Latin or Greek, such as "vastus lateralis" meaning a large muscle to the lateral side. We learn that we must discuss the findings on "radiographs" and never "x-rays." The latter only correctly describes the beam that generates the image, rather than the image itself. Doctorspeak ignores the fact that hardly anyone in the lay public knows what "radiographs" means until you teach them that the term refers to the images they call "x-rays."

I don't mean to argue for the triumph of casual language over specific vocabulary. The vernacular should not rule simply because it is easily understood. Precision and accuracy are important in communication within any field.

As with any new language, immersion is an effective method of learning this Doctorspeak. However, few will practice in similar immersion after completion of their medical degree. Beyond radiologists and pathologists, most physicians will spend much more time interacting with a medically uneducated patient population than they will with other physicians. Immersion teaches the language of medicine, but skimps on the skills of translation. Medical schools and residency training programs rarely, if ever, teach this critical translation directly.

During medical school, I found it enlightening to try to explain to my wife the things I learned. I generally enjoyed more learning about her day than talking about what had consumed the balance of mine, but we tried to be consistent in this exercise. It was very instructive to me. It was instructive because it was difficult. My wife may have higher educational achievement and be "smarter than the average bear," but I still found myself stumbling to get her through the kernels of truth I had learned in a given day.

Much of what I had learned any day was useful only for the moment, or as a foundation for later principles. The key was sorting through this information and communicating the central points to her. I think I got better with practice and time. I doubt that I ever considered at the time that I was practicing for my patients, but I was. I was learning translation.

Turning it Over

Throughout secondary, collegiate and medical education, I felt that the best teachers could deftly bring my focus to the critical points in any concept. I now shoulder the responsibility of teaching my patients as their physician. No longer do physicians hold an exclusive monopoly on medical knowledge. Patients usually have access to as much information as physicians via the Internet and other media. I need to help focus a patient's thinking on what is known, what is unknown, and what is important. Patients must learn how confidently that knowledge can be applied to their case and what the critical differences are between treatment options available to them. I must help them appreciate the aspects of their decisions which uncertainty frankly bungles. I wish I had the time and communication skills needed to cover well all these points with each patient, but I do my best to attempt it.

That is the process of shared decision-making. If I have educated a patient well, I should not fear their choices. I should not offer an option with which I am very uncomfortable, unless I do so with my discomfort clearly outlined and a plan for referral to another provider made available.

Too often, when physicians give patients choices, they are like parents letting a toddler choose between royal blue and navy blue socks. They want the child to feel he is making a choice. They don't want his socks not to match. They pull the two sock pairs out from the drawer and set them before him, knowing that it doesn't really matter which of them he chooses.

The other way that a physician offers a shadow of shared decision-making to patients is to set up straw men options. These are options the physician doesn't really consider options at all. All the reasons why the straw men are not worthy of selection are enumerated, knocking each down in turn. Finally, the physician offers a single, preferred option as the graceful resolution to the void left by the fallen straw men.

"All I'm sure of is that I want one operation, rather than many," Jack stated, with some finality in his voice.

Jack was the widowed father of three young girls. Susan, my patient and his youngest daughter, was five years old. She had almost completed her pre-operative chemotherapy and was approaching the time for surgery to remove the tumor. I usually perform the rebuilding of a limb during the same surgery that removes the tumor. Her age introduced significant challenges to this rebuilding part. Reconstruction of the bones and joints removed with tumors also being treated with aggressive chemotherapy always presents challenges in terms of healing and recovery. When the bone to be reconstructed also needs to retain the capacity to double in size as the patient continues skeletal growth, additional challenges pile on. One cannot predictably avoid the need for repeat reconstructive surgeries during the expected skeletal growth of a five-year-old child.

Alternatives to reconstruction of the bone include amputation above the level of the tumor or a modified type of amputation, called rotationplasty. In rotationplasty, I remove the tumor, then shorten and rotate the leg, attaching the bottom of the tibia to the top of the femur. The backward ankle functions as the knee and the foot itself as the lower leg. Rotationplasty patients use prosthetics similar to those used for below-knee amputations. Surgeons perform few rotationplasties in the United States, but many more in Canada and Europe. They offer physical function equal to or better than most bone reconstructive options, but require ongoing use of a prosthetic limb. For very young children, rotationplasties or amputations provide the only options with a high likelihood of a single operation.

Susan's tumor was in the middle of the bone. Many surgeons would prefer to fill the large gap with a bone graft as a transplant from a deceased donor. We call such grafts "allografts." In our discussion it became increasingly clear that Jack and Susan wanted a rotationplasty, rather than an allograft reconstruction. Usually it is the other way around, but they were trying to convince me that rotationplasty was Susan's best option. They chose between one option that would be surgically finished after one surgery but would require prosthetic use for life, and a second option that would require at least one additional significant surgery later in growth. Jack and Susan accepted the physical uncertainties of prosthetic use to avoid the medical uncertainties of additional surgeries.

My own initial prejudice interested me the most. I had mentioned rotationplasty while proceeding through my typical discussion of limb-salvage with Jack and Susan. I considered amputation and rotationplasty more as options that must be mentioned for a complete list. I am ashamed to say, but they were nearly straw men. I never imagined that Jack would pay such close attention to them. When the discussion caught on rotationplasty, I had to reconsider it myself. Of course, it really is an option. It is a very good option, although rarely pursued by parents or patients. It is so uncommonly chosen whenever another option short of amputation exists that I don't think I expected Jack to consider it seriously. His unexpected focus on that option --- my own preferred option for many other situations --- forced me to stop and really weigh out the critical comparisons and contrasts to the allograft option.

I made lists in my mind. The length of recovery differs appreciably. An allograft would require non-weight-bearing in Susan's lower-limb during healing, which ranges from six months to four times that. For a five-year-old, non-weight-bearing would probably entail wheelchair use for that entire duration. Prosthetic use for a lifetime following rotationplasty is no trifle either, though, even if one initiates walking more quickly following surgery. Allografts also incur more short-term complications in terms of infections and failures of bone healing. The problems of prosthetic fitting probably balance these out reasonably well. Finally, I settled on the greatest challenge I feel each option invites.

"I guess you have to choose which option worries you the least," I began. "Which challenge do you more want to avoid? With rotationplasty, you will have to coach a teenage girl through the emotions of having a backwards foot, the wearing of a prosthetic limb and all the body-image, self-perception, and peer-perception issues that come along with those. Studies show that she will have the same expected rate for marriage and childbearing, or gross measures for adult social success, but even ultimate social success will not erase the challenges of adolescence. With an allograft reconstruction, Susan will have a more normal appearing limb, but will have to plan on another major surgery during the pre-teen and/or teenage years."

In the end, Jack and Susan together opted for the rotationplasty, as much as a five-year-old can really participate in such a decision. I gave them a few weeks' leeway to change their minds about it. They didn't waver. Jack may be a braver man than most, willing to face such difficult issues with Susan in her teenage years as a single father. A daughter's puberty alone frightens most fathers out of their wits. Or, perhaps, rather than brave in his parental role, he was more frightened of hospitals and surgery than emotions. I didn't ask the details of his wife's relatively recent passing. It might have played a role in his dislike of hospitals.

Whatever his reasoning was, it was his decision. I did the very best I could to advise him, to educate him about possibilities and uncertainties. I even made sure that Jack understood that he was choosing a very rarely chosen option, even one that some surgeons wouldn't offer.

Many surgeons would call me crazy even to attempt such shared decision-making with my patients. Sometimes, we so monomaniacally focus on the technical success of our treatment interventions that we forget the decisions made in undertaking such major interventions.

Given the uncertainties intrinsic to such technical successes, I want to be sure that I face them with patients. Otherwise, I will necessarily default into parceling out uncertainties into those that I will silence and others that patients will live with. Some would argue --- and they may be correct --- that if we attempted the allograft, it failed, and Susan ended up with a rotationplasty as a back-up salvage, she would have lost nothing; she would still have the rotationplasty and would have gained the "due process" of trying everything to save the limb. I would rather give her due process in the decision ahead of time insofar as I am able.

Consent in Form

Even if a patient doesn't choose her treatment after a physician teaches her the options, she at least must consent to it after being informed of what it will entail. The concept of informed consent seriously complicates the communication of the uncertainties of treatment, often forcing real shared decision-making back into the shadows.

The history of informed consent is reasonably short. Courts, rather than clinic rooms, and judges, rather than physicians and patients, codified informed consent as legal rather than ethical doctrine. In 1972, *Canterbury v. Spence* was one of the first court rulings even to mention a patient's right to decide for or against a given medical intervention after learning about its risks.[4] Many previous cases discussed the right to information, but this ruling specifically created the necessity for risk disclosure on the "occasion for decision as to whether a particular treatment procedure is to be undertaken."

What most fascinates me about the case, though, is that we completely lose the sense it makes in the court when we consider its medical context. Mr. Canterbury sued Dr. Spence when, one day after a laminectomy procedure, or surgery to remove some of the small protective (and/or impinging) bony elements from behind the spinal cord and nerve roots, he fell out of bed, resulting in paralysis. The court ruled that Dr. Spence should have warned of the possibility of paralysis following laminectomy.

While paralysis can be caused by an intra-operative problem during the course of laminectomy, does this really have anything to do with the freak accident that followed the successful surgery, rendering Mr. Canterbury paralyzed? He fell out of bed, after waking up from a surgery that had caused no paralysis. Thus, rather than from an *ethical* duty to inform patients such that they can choose interventions wisely, informed consent arose from the *legal* duty to warn patients of every possible untoward event that may transpire during or even after surgery.

I don't mean to criticize the legal forum for these definitions. Rather, the world of medicine failed to teach itself of these necessities from a pre-legal, moral standpoint. Courts had to step into the gap medicine had left wide open.

Nearly every surgical or procedural intervention performed in American health care requires documentation of a discussion between the physician and patient of the treatment plan and the risks involved. Sometimes I ask myself for whom I initiate this conversation. Is it for the patient? Or is it rather for attorneys, risk management departments of insurance companies, and the ladies and gentlemen of juries? Its content, particularly its documented content, has more to do with legalities than the patient-doctor relationship.

Herman Melville, the great American novelist, describes a surgical consent discussion of sorts in a lesser-known novel called *Whitejacket*. While Melville wrote this many decades prior to the common use of informed consent in medical and surgical practice in the United States, the imagery he creates still fits.[5] A ship's surgeon explains the amputation he intends to perform on a seaman who sustained a gunshot to the thigh. Reviewing in grotesque detail the painful exercise he plans for the seaman's limb, the surgeon waxes long-winded in his flamboyant lecture to the captivated entire crew.

After mere initiation of the discussion, the patient loses consciousness from dismay over the anticipated discomforts. The fainting of the patient in no way tempers the surgeon's enthusiasm for the discussion. He performs the amputation itself also before the crew and with a grand flourish. After the procedure, the lecture resumes while assistants whisk the patient back to the ship's galley for recovery. Only when these attendants return and announce that the seaman has expired does the lecture draw to a close.

Melville intends satirical humor in this scene. Without subtlety, he pokes fun at how intolerable and ineffective medical treatments were at the time. He portrays the ridiculous self-importance of a practitioner of a crude and unsuccessful art. While our art may have improved, the scene still today satirizes modern informed consent discussions with patients.

I feel more like an attorney than a physician in some of these discussions. Every surgeon takes great effort to explain how unlikely it is that someone will die from a freak anaesthetic complication or sudden, unstoppable exsanguination by hemorrhage, or no patient would ever sign the documentation after such a discussion. We express in spoken verbiage something similar to the list of provisos and exceptions that you expect when signing a 10-page mortgage contract, or when clicking "I agree" at the end of a software terms-and-conditions explanation. Legally, we have to have these conversations, but I fear that they don't meet our ethical obligation to explain what patients can and cannot expect.

Some patients and their families try to end even these consent discussions prematurely, not wanting to hear the morbid possibilities of which I must warn them. It amazes me sometimes how frightened patients and families can be about the one-in-fifty-thousand scale chances that we discuss in these legal consent conversations. Do they forget that in the process of discussing whether or not to pursue surgery at all we have just covered much more frequent uncertainties, many much more ominous in character, only a few minutes prior?

Does a miniscule risk of death by freak accident under anaesthesia really weigh more heavily than a fifty-fifty chance that the surgery will not even accomplish its stated goal? Their protests cause me to doubt how well I really have educated them during the preceding discussions and shared decisions. Legalities may require informed consent, and physician and patient can sign it when complete, but physician-educated, patient-directed decision-making it is not.

I fear that many physicians and surgeons hide behind this legal and technical informed-consent discussion rather than actually educating their patients and shouldering the real uncertainties together. We may not all develop Nathan Rich's quiet confidence as a patient educator and advocate, but we can strive for it.

Communicating some treatment uncertainties is no more complicated (and just as unsatisfying) as simply acknowledging that the best physicians can do is guess and hopefully err on the side of safety for the patient. For more subtle judgments, where practitioners spread across a range of opinions, a physician can let patients know where he fits along the spectrum. Patients and physicians can only reduce treatment if we are willing to enroll in trials that will teach us more about our decisions. I would prescribe a strong dose of less salesmanship and more honesty for physician conversations about treatment with patients. When physicians fail to try to educate their patients about the treatment uncertainties they unavoidably face, they commit the entire experience to physician silence and potentially patient suffering.

Starting Your Conversation. . . .

Picking Poison

Principle: We will either over-treat or under-treat every ailment. For very dangerous conditions we are very wary to reduce the severity of our over-treatments, for fear of failing to win as often.

Ask your physician: Will we slowly ramp up our treatment until symptoms resolve or hit it hard then try to scale back later? Will we be able to scale back later?

Marginal Circumstance

Principle: Physicians will vary along a spectrum for their field with regard to their opinion about any matter. Most know how their opinions fall along that spectrum.

Ask your physician: Where do you stand along the spectrum in your field on this topic?

Sidestep

Principle: Physicians, especially surgeons, struggle to enroll patients in trials because they have difficulty acknowledging doubts about the value of what they can offer, which doubts are necessary to permit randomization between two treatment groups.

Ask your physician: Are there any clinical trials available for my condition?

Dosing Nonsense

Principle: A physician fearing a patient's rejection, may withhold uncomfortable truths.

Ask your physician: If I were your neighbor, to whom would you send me to sort out my problem?

Intrepid

Principle: Courage can enable some of the most difficult decisions to be made even in the midst of great uncertainty. Physicians must be brave to admit that they don't know the right answer.

Ask your physician: Will you let me know when we reach the unknowable parts of my case?

Turning it Over

Principle: Physicians and patients can only share decisions after physicians have explained options and taught the patients about the salient differences between the options.

Ask your physician: Can you teach me how you think through my available options?

Consent in Form

Principle: Informed consent in its legal form too often replaces a physician's ethical responsibility to advise patients about their available options.

Ask your physician: Besides the very rare complications about which you legally must and have already told me, what potentially bad results of this treatment do you consider important enough to weigh in actually deciding to recommend it?

Part Three: Prognosis

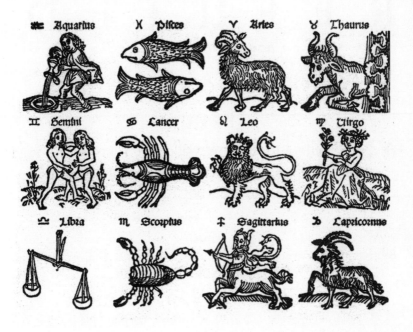

Physick Refined.

The common ERRORS therein

REFUTED,

And the whole ART

Reformed & Rectified:

BEING

A New Rise and Progress of PHYLOSOPHY and MEDICINE, for the Destruction of Diseases and Prolongation of Life.

Written

By that most Learned, Famous, Profound, and Acute Phylosopher, and Chymical Physitian,

John Baptista Van Helmont,

Toparch or Governor, in *Morede, Royenborch, Oorschot, Pellines,* &c.
And now faithfully rendred into *English,* in tendency to a common good, and the increase of true Science ; By

J. C. Sometime of *M. H. Oxon.*

LONDON,
Printed for *Lodowick Loyd,* and are to be sold at his Shop next the *Castle* in *Cornhill.* 1662.

KNOWING THE END FROM THE BEGINNING

pH-balanced

The young surgeon crumpled into a chair, exhausted. She had just wheeled her patient into the ICU bay after hours in the OR. The anesthesiologist and chief ICU physician exchanged notes, hovering over the ventilator settings and intravenous drips. The nursing team busied itself with organizing the forest of intravenous poles and transferring wires from portable monitors at the foot of the transportation cart to large screens suspended from articulated beams that floated over the patient's head.

From mid-calf on her green scrub pants to her plastic clogs, the surgeon was drenched in the patient's blood. She and her team had worked on the yet-unnamed patient, Trauma Number 1519, almost all night.

By report, Mr. 1519 had failed to pay for some services he solicited from two women. One of them then shot him with her handgun at very close range. The bullet went through his hand held up in defense, broke his jaw bone, traversed his neck, tore through his lung on one side, ripping open the major pulmonary artery where it left the heart, dove through the liver, and punched a few holes in loops of the small intestine before coming to rest deep in the abdomen.

Neither the enumeration of his many injuries from a single bullet nor the enormity and depravity of the circumstances leading to his being shot was astonishing to anyone considering the case of Trauma Number 1519. Nonetheless, he had been the central topic of discussion in the surgical ICU for hours before we even met him. As with all high-level trauma team activations, paramedics had apprised the ICU team of his situation since the ambulance picked him up and headed to our emergency room. Since his arrival in the trauma bay downstairs, we had followed by computer the parts of his case for which we would eventually assume responsibility. We knew that once the trauma surgeons had patched up everything that was absolutely critical, they would turn his care over to us for additional tuning up, or resuscitation.

Resuscitation consists of providing intravenous fluids and blood transfusions to enable the heart and lungs to deliver oxygen through the vessels to the tissues. When in shock from injury, acute blood loss, or both, the body cannot effectively deliver oxygen to the organs and tissues. In the absence of oxygen, organs don't immediately die. Cells have the capacity, albeit limited, to survive in the absence of oxygen. During this oxygen-free metabolism, cells produce abundant lactic acid. The lactic acid level slowly builds in the blood stream.

As the team who would ultimately manage this resuscitation for Trauma Number 1519, we attended to the lab values of a variety of blood tests drawn in the ER and then the OR. The most rapid feedback available comes from what are called arterial blood gas (ABG) specimens. Available within minutes, these give a sense of where things are. ABGs offer a few different numbers to follow. Most important to his resuscitation (or the returning of his bodily tissues to oxygen-using metabolism) and thus most important to us were his lactic acid level itself and the pH of his arterial blood.

Once basic circulation stabilizes and begins to support itself, the body can begin to deliver oxygen to reverse this lactic acid buildup. A high lactic acid level itself ultimately brings about the demise of many trauma victims. Human physiology very tightly regulates acid-base balance, or pH, in the bloodstream and tissues. Most mammals biologically maintain the pH very close to 7.4, or just to the basic side of dead neutral (pH 7.0). Straying far in either direction on this logarithmic scale will cause most of the protein enzymes that drive metabolic physiology to stop functioning. Because the generation of lactic acid itself requires functioning enzymes, there are theoretical limits to how acidic (or low in number) the pH can get before the cells die and stop producing more acid.

"Six-point-five!" The chief resident on-call had exclaimed when the values from the first ABG from the ER flashed onto our screen. "No way. You would die before your body could even produce enough lactic acid to get your pH down to 6.5. It just can't be correct. But one thing is for sure: if Mr. 1519 has a pH anywhere near 6.5, he will not survive long enough to fill one of our beds tonight. I can't believe that he really got there, but there's no way they'll bring him back from pH 6.5 if he did get there."

Levels of 7.0 or 6.9 represent extremely severe acidosis.

None of us watching the numbers roll in that night will ever know if 6.5 was indeed correct, but the pH corrected slowly enough from that point that we suspect it was at least close. Just as remarkably, they got him through the night in the OR, patched up his neck and chest injuries, and delivered him into our care before he showed any clear signs other than his pH that were strictly incompatible with life. We remained convinced that the heroic surgical effort to staunch his pulmonary arterial hemorrhage would fail in the end. "Surviving" on a respirator with blood replacement pouring into his veins might do for a few hours, but his body would certainly declare failure by the middle of the next day. He had, after all, had a pH of 6.5.

We were wrong. Mr. 1519 did survive the morning and afternoon and evening, even to the next day, when another surgery patched up the intestinal and liver injuries. He kept surviving until the surgeons had the opportunity to patch up everything, believe it or not. We didn't believe it when, toward the end of the month, he managed to breathe for himself off the ventilator.

He even woke up enough that he could tell us a real name. When he left the ICU for a step-down unit, we guessed that he hadn't achieved his baseline psychological/neurological status, but he was alive.

Even without an inspiring personal story, Mr. 1519 broke the rules.

He survived what we thought was an impossible, not merely improbable, circumstance.

Trauma number 1519 taught us once again that we don't necessarily know what we think we know, especially when we try to predict the future from the present.

Dead Man's Bluff

The word prognosis derives from the Greek and means knowing ahead of time. You might argue that Mr. 1519 beat the impossible odds of our initial prognosis because so many skilled providers brought to bear so many life-saving technologies. I don't personally think that can explain away recovery from a pH of 6.5, but it is a valid argument. Medicine might tweak impossibility all the time, by sheer force of will and Herculean effort. If that prognosis failed because we worked diligently to change it, can we predict better when we choose not to intervene?

What happens when poor prognosis drives a care team to stop trying, to give up on a patient's capacity for a return to function? Do our predictions function better in a less manipulated circumstance?

Care teams occasionally abandon care provision to chance when poor prognosis prompts a family to withdraw life-support from a critically ill patient in an ICU. A patient on a ventilator, or breathing machine that inflates the lungs through a tube placed into the windpipe, depends on this machine for life about as much as a human can. When the team judges that dependent patient to have little chance of meaningful recovery, the family may choose "terminal extubation." The care team removes the tube from the trachea and therefore the patient's connection with the ventilator. Tube removal fits the "extubation" half of the term. "Terminal" communicates the sense that the decision is both final and will result in death.

Some families and physicians worry that terminal extubation is tantamount to murder. Is removing necessary life support the same as taking life? Maybe. We are not that skilled at achieving certainty in the "necessary" determination.

A recent observational study reviewed a single hospital's experience with terminal extubation over a duration of time.[1] The hospital's physicians had performed twenty-one such extubations during the recorded period. Three patients had survived not only minutes and hours but days --- long enough to be discharged from the hospital, and not via the morgue. This one-in-seven rate of someone beating impossible odds signifies that the odds must not have been as impossible as predicted. Perhaps that particular hospital is especially poor at generating prognoses for ventilator-dependent patients. I doubt it. The practitioners there are probably about as poorly skilled at prognosis as physicians are everywhere.

Perhaps each of the three died within days or weeks of leaving the hospital. I don't know the details. In one rather publicized case of survival to discharge after terminal extubation, the patient lived for nine additional years. National news agencies brought focus to Karen Ann Quinlan's case in the 1970s, when her family requested extubation, but the hospital initially refused. Right-to-die groups rallied around her cause. A judge ordered that the hospital comply with the family's wishes. The hospital performed the terminal extubation. Karen didn't wake up after terminal extubation, but she did survive. She survived until a pneumonia, left untreated, took the remaining vestiges of her tube-fed, persistent vegetative state of life in the mid 1980s.

More extreme than survival after terminal extubation, some patients survive --- or at least regain a heart rhythm --- after the declaration of death itself. Since the 1980s, medical journals have reported more than 25 cases of what were termed Lazarus syndrome.[2] The name refers to the Biblical account of Jesus' friend, rising from death at His command. We more technically refer to Lazarus syndrome as spontaneous return of circulation after failed cardiopulmonary resuscitation (CPR). After initiation of CPR, the care provider frequently assesses for any return of pulse or breathing while continuing to support at least some circulation of oxygen-carrying blood to the brain. The physically demanding chest compressions and forced ventilation of the lungs by mouth-to-mouth or bag-and-mask don't continue indefinitely. After some duration, the code, or CPR session, will be "called," signs of life checked one more time, and death declared in their confirmed absence. Lazarus syndrome is the later return of a heart rhythm with or without respiration.

Some have speculated that these post-death-declaration reawakenings come about due to relaxation of the CPR-overinflated chest cavity. As the chest relaxes, the blood it blocked from returning to the heart is allowed in; the subtle electrical charges generated can stimulate the heart to beat again.

Few in this elite group of the reawakened will return to home, have friends over for dinner, and tell about their near-death --- or perhaps past-death --- experiences. Some will. The existence of these cases tells me of the limits of our ability to predict. After a trajectory of care was abandoned to let nature take its course and that natural course was deemed complete, the prognosis undid itself.

Physicians struggle sufficiently with diagnosis --- the assessment of what has already happened in the immediate or distant past --- and treatment decision-making, the determination of what should happen in the present. Most will wisely shy away from bold projections of the future. Medicine cannot escape the future entirely, though. To some extent, every medical intervention includes the hope that it will derail a train headed for an unfavorable future. When mortality specifically hangs in the balance, we predict only with extreme caution.

There is a Greek myth at the foundation of the medical philosophy that dominates modern medicine in the Western world. The myth emphasizes the danger of tampering with death. Aesculapius, around whose staff you have seen the snakes intertwine, used his surgical arts to prevent the death he not only predicted for his patient, but that Zeus intended. Thwarted in his execution of an intended fate by Aesculapius' medical magic, Zeus turned his thunderbolt on the physician instead.[3] While I assume that his intervention offended most, Aesculapius' daring to make the prediction in the first place might not be so much less offensive.

Fortunately for physicians, death doesn't hang in the balance of every prognosis. Unfortunately, life hangs in most. Although recoveries from not-as-terminal-as-initially-suspected terminal extubation or Lazarus syndrome are extreme and relatively rare examples, they illustrate how poorly physicians predict the end, even at what appear to be dead-end roads.

The New Math

"The part I'm not comfortable with is this risk for the radiation causing another cancer in the same area." Cindy struggled with my recommendation that she pursue radiation as an added treatment for a tumor I had recently removed from her buttocks.

I agreed with her. "Yes. That is a real chance, no doubt."

"I just cannot imagine how it would feel to go through all this again." Cindy had a very pleasant demeanor but had already proven that anxiety added difficulty to her cancer experience.

She came to see me to evaluate what turned out to be a large soft-tissue sarcoma of the buttocks muscle. This large, high-grade cancer posed a significant threat to her life and limb. She had resigned herself to the deeply invasive surgery I had performed to remove the nearly football-sized mass from her tissues, but she struggled with the need for radiation.

I usually prefer the administration of radiation prior to surgery for removal of the sarcoma. She had flatly refused it at that juncture. I had agreed to proceed with surgery on the condition that if any margin on the final resection was less than a full centimeter, I would as much as insist on radiation to follow the surgery.

I had cut as widely as I could without sacrificing major nerves and vessels. The large tumor had invaded so many tissue planes that I had to remove abundant muscle even to achieve limited margins. The pathologist had judged the margins to be negative, meaning that no tumor touched the planes we had dissected. They were not all greater than a full centimeter in thickness, however.

This negative margin, or layer of normal tissue surrounding the tumor, was sufficiently thick to render Cindy's risk of tumor recurrence in what was left of her buttock to about five percent, *if* she agreed to the radiation I now recommended. If she refused it again, her risk jumped at least to 20 percent, if not twice that. These tumors usually have established tiny satellites in the surrounding tissues. Radiation predictably eradicates such invisible satellite colonies of sarcoma.

"The risk of a radiation-induced secondary sarcoma hovers around 1 percent, as you know," I repeated for her.

"I know, but this first round of cancer has been bad enough, hasn't it?"

I continued, "I don't mean to downplay the possibility of a future cancer bringing new difficulties. In fact, a second cancer in this limb would likely require more drastic surgery, perhaps even amputation. But, . . ."

"Exactly," she interrupted. "I hear the second time is always worse."

"But," I emphasized, "your first time isn't necessarily over yet."

"What do you mean?"

"You cannot have a worse sarcoma in your buttock than you already have had. This was as high-grade and high-risk as any radiation-induced sarcoma could be. A *recurrence* of your particularly nasty first sarcoma would be just as bad as a secondary one. The only difference is that it would likely happen one to two decades sooner.

"You have at least a twenty percent --- and some would say much higher --- chance of your first cancer coming back in the buttock. You can cut that chance down to five percent with a course of radiation. Yes, it costs you a one-percent chance of a second cancer in a decade or two, but the trade-off definitely favors radiation now. Twenty minus fifteen plus one is still six, a lot less than twenty."

Cindy didn't love this math, but I knew of no other way to reason it out for her. I had no doubt about the decision I preferred. But I couldn't predict her future.

I didn't discuss it with Cindy, but while she was making this decision, I had two patients struggling with secondary cancers. Both were much less likely to occur than Cindy's would be. Neither one related to radiation.

One developed a bone sarcoma more than a decade after treatment of a brain tumor in infancy. While Cindy pondered her fate, he lay dying at home. His parents had recently thanked their chemotherapy specialist, who had seen them through both battles, for the years they had enjoyed in between.

My other patient had her bone sarcoma first but was then in the hospital undergoing a bone marrow transplant to treat a secondary leukemia only a year after completion of chemotherapy for her sarcoma. She was actually one of the first bone sarcomas I treated after arriving in Utah. Would I ever have predicted that she would draw that shortest straw? I knew it was there for the drawing. Yet I didn't see that end from the beginning. I only hope her transplant manages to divert her possible end into a beginning.

As much as these two secondary cancers pain my patients and me in the experiences they generate, they are no more painful than would be the return of an inadequately treated cancer in Cindy's case. The prognosis, ephemeral as it may be, matters for the decision-making. We may not have crystal balls stored in the pockets of our white coats, but we must make population-based predictions to guide our decisions in the present. If I predicted that Cindy's risk of a secondary sarcoma from the radiation were fifty percent but it only reduced her chance of a recurrence of her first cancer by 10 percent, I would have to recommend consideration of accepting the small short-term risk in exchange for avoiding the large long-term risk.

In this way, every treatment decision depends on prognosis. The best physicians can offer is number-based predictions of a patient's possible futures. We need these rough predictions to make treatment decisions but cannot really trust them as predictions in and of themselves. The extremes --- and every possibility in between --- remain potential future experiences for the patient.

Catching Curves

Stuart Weinstein is a legend who becomes more legendary the better you know him. As I finished medical school in Baltimore, one of my mentors there advised me to spend as much time around Dr. Weinstein as I possibly could during my anticipated years in residency training at his program.

"Stuart Weinstein has accomplished at least…" --- he paused while counting quickly on his fingers --- "at least nine things, any one of which would have been a great career achievement for an academic orthopaedic surgeon!"

As his wife was my realtor, I met Dr. Weinstein a few weeks before I began my residency training. He and his wife took my wife and me out to dinner after she had shown us a number of housing options. His white hair and quiet manner gave him a distinguished look beyond his actual age.

As we entered the restaurant, someone offered warm greetings to his wife. He smiled sheepishly. "Lynn knows everyone in this town. No one has any idea what my name is."

I appreciated his humility. He realized that fame in the world of academic orthopaedic surgery wasn't fame that mattered in social circles. This didn't trouble him one bit.

Once I started working in his department, I learned quickly that Dr. Weinstein approached pediatric patients and their parents with the same humble --- almost shy --- demeanor and care that he offered to colleagues and residents. Most patients and their families clearly adored having him as their surgeon. He took this role and its responsibility very seriously.

During my first year in the program, Dr. Weinstein added a tenth major career accomplishment. Orthopaedic surgeons rarely author an article in *JAMA*, or the *Journal of the American Medical Association*.[4] *JAMA*, one of the highest-impact general medical journals, usually focuses its publications on large randomized controlled drug trials. In fact, as best I can ascertain, an orthopaedic surgeon has authored a *JAMA* paper only a handful of other times in the last two decades.

Dr. Weinstein's article didn't report on some large, multicenter, randomized controlled trial of a new life-saving drug; it reported on a follow-up study of no intervention at all. The study had tracked at 50 years a group of patients who had received no surgical treatment for scoliosis when diagnosed during adolescence. Obviously, even with white hair, Dr. Weinstein hadn't seen these patients initially himself. He had taken over the care of some of them on the retirement of his teacher, mentor and senior partner, Ignacio V. Ponseti. Those patients whom Dr. Weinstein hadn't met were also contacted. Ultimately, a large group of Dr. Ponseti's patients from the 1940s and early 1950s came back to the clinic to fill out questionnaires and have spine radiographs obtained.

Dr. Ponseti had begun his practice not so long after surgery emerged as a viable treatment paradigm for non-life-threatening diagnoses. The invention of anaesthesia rendered surgery tolerable, and sterile technique improved its survivability to much better than half, but it was the antibiotics developed during the Second World War that really broadened its scope. A number of surgical interventions common now were yet undertaken dubiously in the 1940s.

Dr. Ponseti approached the practice of pediatric orthopaedic surgery in that environment of palpable uncertainty with the added skepticism of a scientist. He judged some interventions that other surgeons had quickly adopted to be ill-conceived, short-term solutions for long-term problems.

And Dr. Ponseti knew the difference between short- and long-term problems. Before moving to Iowa City, he had pursued his own orthopaedic training as a field surgeon in the Spanish Civil War. Without antibiotics available, he and his mentor had shown that casting and repeated surgical debridements of open fractures (broken bones that came through the skin at the time of injury) resulted in fewer deaths. Scoliosis didn't dance with death as did those battlefield open fractures. The only short-term deaths from scoliosis of which Ponseti was aware were disastrous complications of surgeries gone wrong. No, scoliosis was a slow diagnosis, not meriting surgery in his opinion.

If Dr. Ponseti offered no fix for the curved spine, how did he catalogue so many new patients in such a short time? Patients with scoliosis came to him because his clinic was the only option for scoliosis care in Iowa. Scoliosis weighed on the public consciousness because others publicized new treatments for it.

As soon as the technology became available to straighten curved spines, some surgeons employed it to do so; the world of medicine already "knew" that curved spines, left unstraightened, would be a problem later in life. By this point in the book, it shouldn't surprise you to hear that while the world of medicine *thought* it knew just that, it had deeply studied nothing of the sort. No, that knowledge in any tractable form wouldn't arrive until 50 years after surgeons started fusing spines. Technical innovations permitting the intervention to correct scoliosis prompted more regimented diagnosis of the condition in the first place.

It isn't that surgeons only recognized scoliosis after surgery became available for it; it's more that they only pursued and carefully recorded diagnosis of it on a large scale after it had an available intervention. Ideally they would have randomized patients to the new intervention or standard non-operative therapy, but such study methods were not broadly recognized in that era. The first randomized controlled trial of any type was reported in 1948. Only Dr. Ponseti's skepticism that scoliosis fusions were helpful kept him from operating on the patients that ended up in the study. Had it not been for his skepticism, we might not yet know what problems or lack thereof scoliosis fusions hoped to prevent.

Because Dr. Ponseti had stored spine radiographs obtained from the study patients during their adolescence, analyses could be made to develop better predictions of scoliosis progression over time from measurements of those early radiographs. Some spine curvature measurements during adolescence correlated well with worsening of the scoliosis after skeletal maturity. Curves below these thresholds changed little even over the subsequent fifty years. These data from 50-year follow-up patients validated some and refuted other prediction schemes that shorter-duration studies had previously developed.

Such predictions of scoliosis progression from clinical and radiographic measurements guide decisions regarding if and when to intervene. The prognosis subgroups of scoliosis defined by these measurements therefore become distinct diagnoses, meriting distinct therapies. In many ways, the prognosis for a given scoliosis *is* the diagnosis.

While a detailed prognosis of the future from features of a child's or adolescent's clinical situation is desirable, it remains a correlation, not a hard fact. As uncertain as they still are, such prognoses provide our best identification of treatment-worthy problems.

Prognoses may be no more than diagnoses in the same way that diagnoses are really no more than prognoses. Remember that the meaning of a diagnosis was primarily couched in the predicted natural course of disease that some treatment would hope to alter.

Straight-up

Notably, this *JAMA* scoliosis study wasn't Stuart Weinstein's first 50-year follow-up study of a pediatric orthopaedic condition. He performed similar studies for developmental hip dysplasia, club foot, and others. Many pediatric orthopaedic conditions appear initially not as immediate problems, but as noted radiographic abnormalities or bodily deformities. Intervention aims at altering the long-term prognosis, rather than fixing an immediate problem. Patients might often willingly live with a slight crookedness of spine or limb if they knew that it wouldn't lead to disabling pain and loss of function later in life.

Identification of a problem worthy of treatment or a poor prognosis clearly linked to specific features of an otherwise asymptomatic condition only barely begins the work of knowing. We might call these features risk factors for the long-term unfavorable outcome. The question then becomes whether or not these risk factors are modifiable. Can any intervention address those risk factors in a way that ameliorates the prognosis? Then follows the question, which of the broad array of potential interventions most effectively improves the long-term prognosis?

Most remarkable of the *JAMA* scoliosis study results was that these patients, 50 years beyond their diagnosis, were generally doing well. The back and breathing problems that many physicians once speculated would result from untreated scoliosis had disabled very few of the study patients. How can an intervention meaningfully improve on that tolerable result of no treatment at 50 years?

Evaluating the correction of the generally mild difficulties that follow by 50 years the diagnosis of scoliosis requires another 50-year study. One finds few long-term follow-up studies from the early surgical fusion treatments of scoliosis. All available studies were performed in Sweden. None spans 50 years. The overall functional outcome of these patients isn't dramatically better than Dr. Weinstein's long-term follow-up of Dr. Ponseti's untreated patients.[5] Many potential biases may influence the small appreciable differences in results. The studies come from different centers. Maybe Iowans are tougher than Swedes, reflecting a shift in patient-reported function; maybe only the worst patients underwent surgery.

To complicate the situation further, no one still performs any of the early scoliosis interventions for which long-term results are available. Scoliosis fusion surgeries have "improved" since then in a couple of major ways. Will these technical "improvements" translate into improved function at 50 years? Your prognosis is as good as mine. I hope they will. I even think they will. Whatever they accomplish, they illustrate a major challenge to understanding the long-term effects of conditions and our treatments. "Improvements" tend to be new technologies designed to improve upon previously available technologies. Unfortunately, not all improvements step forward. Some step sideways. Some step backward.

A few clinicians favor nihilism after reading a 50-year follow-up with good results of no treatment. These might suggest that it is in spite of his study, but Stuart Weinstein continues to perform massive spine fusion surgeries for adolescents with scoliosis. Some weeks, he performs four in a week. What did the study teach him?

"The data back up what I have supposed for a long time," he will tell critics. "I now have facts to discuss with my patients, rather than just suppositions. I want them to understand that pursuing scoliosis surgery is their choice. They would still live a productive, functional life without it in most cases. The main difference in many cases is appearance. Don't misunderstand, that isn't a dismissal. Appearance matters immensely to the teenagers this condition afflicts. I don't think it is wrong to straighten the scoliotic spine. What is wrong is threatening people that not pursuing surgery will lead to disabling back pain and respiratory compromise. I never did tell patients that, but some did. As usual, data simply keep us honest."

Data don't remove uncertainty or dictate what the exactly right thing to do is. Data can teach physicians what to teach their patients.

Hammers and Nails

I can easily forgive the medical world of Dr. Ponseti's early practice years for failing to randomize patients between surgical fusion
and no-treatment groups. I might appropriately argue that such
study designs cannot practically render fifty-year results anyway. At
least Dr. Ponseti was skeptical and kept good records, permitting
some measure of the prognosis fifty years later.

The general approach of identifying and studying treatment-
worthy conditions only after treatments become available didn't
limit itself to the period of elective surgical discovery following
the Second World War and the advent of antibiotics. Much more
recently, many proverbial nails to hit have only been identified
after a hammer was in hand. Diagnoses continue to emerge after
therapies are discovered. Each begs the question: what is the prognosis of each new diagnosis? How can it change with treatment?

Just a few years ago, a new version of an old technique was
described to reorient the hip socket in young adults. Soon after its
sudden popularity for the rare circumstance of hip dysplasia that
missed earlier diagnosis, reports began to crop up in the literature
of previously unrecognized conditions that *needed* this treatment.
Many experienced surgeons considered some of these newly recognized conditions as resulting from a ridiculous scramble to find
nails to fit the newfound hammer.

I recall comments such as, "If all these people have such disas-
ters impending in their hips, why did I never see them coming to
my office over 30 years of hip surgery practice?" While I generally
shared the skepticism, I must admit that medicine has never been
skilled at recognizing entities for which it wasn't looking. If there
really are newly recognized diagnoses or grouped features of hip
anatomy that can be addressed by seriously invasive new surgical
techniques, what do these newly recognized disease states mean?
What is their prognosis?

Most surgeons who provide variations on the new techniques
consider withholding such available treatments from their patients
as base treachery. As touching as their patient advocacy may be,
before we can even begin to address the uncertainty of their treat-

ment interventions, we must know what they are actually treating. What prognoses of these new diagnoses do they hope to avert? If every clinician capable of diagnosing the problem or predicting a poor prognosis immediately changes it with a treatment intervention, how can we ever know what the prognosis really was?

Another hip condition has followed that exact history. We know no more about the prognosis of untreated Legg-Calvé-Perthes disease than we did in the days of Drs. Legg, Calvé, and Perthes, a century ago. Almost every reported case series follows up patients who received some intervention. For Legg-Calvé-Perthes disease, all suspect that the natural history must not be good, but no one really knows. We have never witnessed the fulfillment of this poor prognosis from untreated disease in a large series.

For these new hip diagnoses, will we have to wait 50 years to know their prognoses? Will we even have a chance of knowing then? If we have any chance at all, we will depend on the graces of one extraordinarily busy but skeptical surgeon who is now quietly accruing patients whom he dissuades from seeking such interventions. Who will be my generation's Ignacio V. Ponseti? In this age of abundant information and misinformation, how will this new Ponseti convince his patients not to pursue the treatments they want under another pair of hands? They will have more than one choice of hip clinic. We will never know the end from this beginning unless we prepare to measure the end from the beginning. We might then better predict at least the future's future.

Starting Your Conversation. . . .

pH Balanced
Principle: Even when Medicine thinks recovery from a circumstance is impossible, it may be wrong.
Ask your physician: What was the biggest positive surprise you have experienced in a case such as mine?

Dead Man's Bluff
Principle: When Medicine thinks a person is dying or already dead, it may be wrong.
Ask your physician: What are the best and worst case scenarios you have seen for patients with my condition?

The New Math
Principle: Even successful treatments may bring unwanted late effects. These long-term risks must be weighed against short-term benefits.
Ask your physician: What long-term risks do we create by this treatment?

Catching Curves
Principle: Knowing the natural history, or the typical course of untreated disease, can powerfully influence decisions made at diagnosis. The expected course really *is* the diagnosis.
Ask your physician: What is the natural history of my condition? How do we know about it?

Straight-up
Principle: The best measure of any treatment also depends on its long-term impact, or how it changes the natural history.
Ask your physician: What is known about the long-term outcomes of this treatment? Are successes durable?

Hammers and Nails

Principle: The hardest thing about diseases that are recognized only after a treatment becomes available for them is that we never learn the undisturbed course of disease that we are hoping to change.

Ask your physician: Has anyone ever diagnosed conditions just like mine, not treated them, and found out what happened?

IMPROVING THE MORTALITY EXPERIENCE

Paying the Bills

Early in the spring of 1674, a man eyed his yellowing skin; he knew that he was dying. He wouldn't reach his 54th birthday, only a week away. Who could have predicted that the massive fire of 1666, which wiped out the residences of eighty percent of Londoners, would destroy his business, leave him impoverished, and lead him to drunken oblivion and liver failure?

Twelve years prior, when he presented his work to King Charles II and the Royal Society, he had specifically studied the timing of death. Compiling 70 years of death and birth statistics, he had detailed the dynamics of the human population in London. The data so impressed King Charles that he had welcomed John Graunt as a charter member of the Royal Society, despite John's decidedly middle-class merchant and tradesman background.[1]

In retrospect, John had to admit that he had had impeccable timing, presenting his findings and theories at one of the first gatherings of the fledgling group. The right group. The right meetings. The right monarch, even. Queen Elizabeth would never have tolerated a tradesman presenting in her court. Neither would Charles I.

Charles II was different from his father, at least wiser. Yes, impeccable timing. Hadn't impeccable been John Graunt's trade?

Haberdashery thrived on the impeccable. The lords and wealthy merchants who spent their gold in John's drapery shop came precisely because he had impeccable taste in cloth and measured out, cut and tailored impeccably fitting suits.

Ironically, the Fates' measuring and cutting his own longevity seemed unconscious of his knack for impeccable timing. What had gone wrong? Was it his growing love of ale? He knew others who drank more; they were not dying. Was he just unlucky? No one could have expected the fire, of course, but the Black Death, a year before it, had decidedly passed over the Graunt household. John had personally missed the plague twice before that, as a boy during the outbreaks in 1625 and 1636. Luckier still, he had weathered the bloody rise and fall of the Commonwealth and Cromwell's Protectorate. No, it could not be luck.

Could John really complain? He knew, better than any perhaps, that he would only miss his expected life span by a bit under a decade.

Of course, my portrayal of his dying thoughts strays deeply into fiction, but what did John Graunt think as he lay dying of liver failure at the age of 53, only 12 years after creating the science of demography from which would later spring epidemiology, public health and actuarial science? Whatever he thought --- and if he were dying of liver failure as history tells us, the thoughts in his bilirubin-pickled brain may have tended more toward the dances of confabulatory purple peacocks than reasoned self-inquiry --- what he was experiencing was both the boon and bane of making predictions using population science. Such predictions only work when averaged across populations, never for individuals.

John Graunt's book, entitled *Natural and Political Observations Made Upon the Bills of Mortality,* presented the first regimented study of birth and death records for a whole population. It reported life tables that recorded the probability of living to any given age. Such tables still function as the medium for the work of life insurance actuaries. Actuaries now generate lifespan predictions with many more complex variables than were available to John Graunt. They use more complicated mathematical calculations than had been conceived in London in 1662 and more powerful computers to

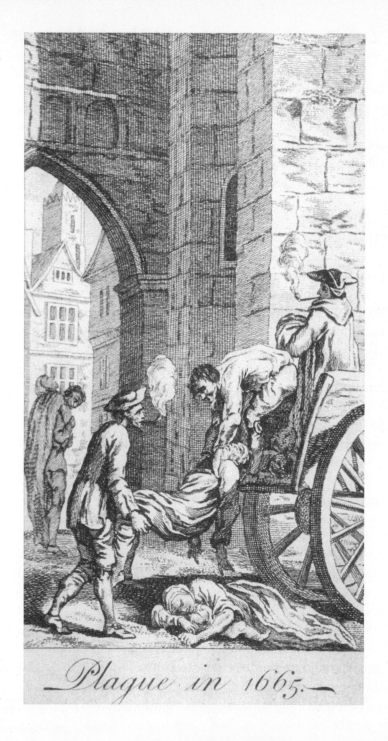

Plague in 1665.

run those calculations than London would see for three hundred years after Graunt's death.

As with all areas of medical uncertainty discussed in this book, humanity also manages prognostic uncertainty by turning to populations. As John Graunt's life exhibits, we can't easily apply populations to individuals as individuals. Nonetheless, it is remarkable what can be known for populations more generally from sub-populations studied.

Gambling

These days, actuarial science has morphed from an intellectual pursuit discussed in the hobnobbing likes of the Royal Society to more of an applied science, discussed behind the closed and locked doors of big business board rooms. Life insurance premiums in the United States total nearly half a trillion dollars each year, with assets owned by life insurance companies many-fold higher.

Despite the depth and breadth of this industry, profit margins remain surprisingly slim, running around 8 percent, most years.[2] While an 8 percent profit margin gives me no reason to feel sorry for the life insurance executives, the relatively small number suggests that industry professionals predict death within an even narrower margin of accuracy. These companies develop algorithms to predict population risks and essentially bet on those predictions, competing with other companies to predict most accurately the longevity of their insured population.

Joseph, a neighbor and friend of mine, earns his living as an actuary for a large life insurance company. He is neither salesman nor scientist. And he isn't a betting man by any stretch of the imagination. Joseph is more of an engineer, a numbers guy. He watches numbers, finds patterns in numbers, thinks in numbers and gives number answers to the business managers who need to make decisions about what policies to sell and how much they should be sold for. Joseph and I chatted recently at a neighborhood event about exactly what his work as an actuary involves.

"The goal is always to improve your mortality experience," he began.

"Say that again." Really, I thought I had misheard him.

"Improve your mortality experience," he repeated.

I laughed. "Can anyone really tell us what his mortality experience is? I mean, who wouldn't want to improve the experience of dying, if we only knew what it actually felt like."

"No, that would be grand, if we could do that. I am afraid that type of life insurance policy would be exorbitantly expensive though. The mortality experience is actuarial lingo indicating the actual deaths your company has been on the hook for in a given subscribing population."

"Even so, you know that I will have to use this for my book."

"It is a funny phrase, I guess," he agreed, with a very mathy look of perplexity. "I'd never really thought of it out of its life insurance context. Nonetheless, I think about it, the mortality experience, from 9 to 5 every day. There is an investment team in the company that tries to optimize the growth of capital resources and predict what growth can be expected over the 20- to 30-year terms we are about to sell, but I mostly crunch numbers on the other side of the hallway. I get new data sets every few weeks for each policy type and each age group and risk group. It's my job to review that mortality experience and see where our formulas predicted well and where they were off in either direction."

"I am guessing that these data sets. . ."

"The mortality experience," he interrupted with a chuckle.

"The mortality experience is pretty large in size, covering large populations," I finished.

"Of course. The larger the better. We're a huge, multi-state company. Our experience is enormous for a given year or even month. We can divide things up by policy, price structures, health variables, age, profession, really any way to parse the data and understand the experience. We want to learn which policies in which populations may be costing us more than anticipated, so that we can raise the price, if needed. We also want to know where we have overestimated the mortality experience, looking for angles to make our pricing more competitive in populations for which we have predicted higher mortality than we actually experienced."

"So these are populations of hundreds and thousands?"

"Oh no. Populations of tens and hundreds of thousands. And they are populations over decades and decades as well. The time factor is really critical."

"So what would you say about a population of one?"

"Laughable. With a population of one, you have a fifty-fifty chance of being wrong in each direction, but you will never be right. A mortality experience of one will always be grossly under- or over-predicted. I literally cannot do my job with a mortality experience of one. Neither can I even apply the mortality experience of a million people over a hundred years to an individual in one year. Our math can tell us nothing about the one. Our predictions come from populations as large as possible and must be applied to populations as large as possible, or they won't be reasonable predictions at all."

"But that's medicine. I only get one patient at a time."

"Well, don't try to predict a mortality experience, whatever you do. Or if you must, at least don't bet money on it."

Working Population

Actuaries aren't the only group who will analyze a mortality experience, though they may be the only ones to call it that positively wry term. Most major health science universities, as well as many state and federal agencies, employ the academically oriented counterparts of actuaries: epidemiologists. Epidemiologists work essentially as public health statisticians, or population scientists. They mathematically review huge population data sets, trying to measure the impact of environmental or health policy or practice changes on the longevity of the population in question.

I recall a particularly insightful presentation I witnessed during my fellowship year of study at the University of Toronto. The researcher visited Toronto from the United Kingdom for a special conference. His epidemiological research focused on the rates of cancer death in populations. He reviewed data from his own country, as well as from both developed and developing nations the world over. His presentation drove home the overarching point that very few health technologies really affect population dynamics in a measurable way, even if one focuses on cancer-specific death. He noted for the audience the timing of the introduction of hormonal treatment for breast carcinoma. As much as this is considered by many to be one of the most significant cancer advances in recent history, the blip it produced in cancer death statistics for the United States was only barely discernible on a greatly magnified small region of the chart.

In stark contrast, he showed how the rise of smoking among men or women in a nation was followed quite strictly by a massive increase in cancer-specific or general death rates in the population, lagging about three decades later.[3] This was comparable to (actually exceeding in some cases) the effect of events like civil war in a country, or some of the well-known epidemics through the last century.

Learning from this data, or at least from the epidemiologists smart enough to make this data digestible for the rest of us, is critical. From this data we learn the effects of societal trends and fads, such as smoking. Even this indirect method offers our best way to discern its effects on people. Epidemiology also appropriately humbles health interventionists (read "physicians"). We can observe how little our very best interventions actually affect the populations for whom we give care. Epidemiology emphasizes that avoidance of large scale civil war, avoidance of smoking, and availability of clean water and antibiotics basically purchased most of the improvements in longevity that are appreciated in modern times --- we can almost ignore the medical advances of the latter half of the 20th century!

Such data derives from massive populations. Such data also only best applies to massive populations. Many individuals who pick up the habit of smoking will not die at the predicted 30-year anniversary of their first light-up. *Most* will not, honestly. You can't be sure that you have saved a single patient from early demise by smoking cessation. If you convince a generation to avoid cigarettes, on the other hand, that is a different story. . . .

Just like my friend the actuary, epidemiologists would scoff at application of their data to individuals. We might glean good principles from it, but pure application doesn't work. They would at least insist that their predictions can't hold true for a population of one. They have bigger fish to fry. They gather their data from large populations to influence matters that affect large populations.

For example, epidemiology can inform governmental policy, as policy necessarily affects large populations. Especially when governments control health care resources for a population, epidemiology figures prominently in the allocation of these resources. Such large government-directed health care programs cannot fuss over the one or the exceptions to the rule. Attending to individuals may be a luxury to which wealthy nations aspire. It might even be a politically important move for those writing the policies. The hard-line epidemiologist, however, cannot see the individual in the wash of numbers on her computer screen.

A comparison between the health care systems of the United States and Canada can instruct our understanding of the differences between populations and the individual. I have worked in both systems. I saw positives and negatives in each. Importantly, the two place very different values on populations and individuals.

During the recent health care debate in the United States, politicians quickly pointed out that as much as America spends on health care, we have no better health as a nation.[4] In fact, we have worse. What are we getting in exchange for our largest-in-the-world health expenditures? We *should* question this.

We should also ask the contrary valid question: if health care is so bad in the United States, why do so many Canadians cross their Southern border for their healthcare? For example, the Cleveland Clinic Foundation opened an office in Toronto that helps Canadians organize care in Cleveland. Do the Canadians who head south for healthcare just foolishly look for a place to pay more for less? Maybe, but probably not.

The explanation for both of these oddities has everything to do with populations and individuals. American health care can throw more resources at a single patient than any other place in the world. In many cases, those resources, when applied astutely, will actually accomplish something good for the recipient. Sometimes, application of so many resources will accomplish something that wouldn't be possible from the application of fewer resources. We can only measure such successes in anecdotes and individual experiences, not in populations.

In contrast, a few, very cheap, broadly and centrally governed resources can accomplish a lot more for a population when applied to things that matter to populations, such as prenatal care and smoking cessation programs. Governments that control the healthcare provisions for nations can hire epidemiologists to find out which factors are important to control and then control them. The provincial health systems in Canada do this precisely, and they do it well. The lack of centralized control in U.S. health care makes the management of such population-based issues impossible.

Centralized governmental control of health care resources necessarily sacrifices some individual liberties. Many in the United States place high value on these individual liberties, which matters immensely in the debate. Both systems, or rather the non-system of United States health care and the system-system of Canadian provincial health programs, have merit. Both also have problems. Critically though, one cannot honestly fault a non-system for not systematically controlling population health variables, if it is set up to focus only on individuals. Conversely, one cannot fault the system-system for allowing an individual to get lost in or overlooked by the programs intended for populations.

Politicians and voting citizens, informed by epidemiologists, organize these systems or non-systems. Policies can powerfully affect mortality rates and longevity in a population. Policies have very little power on the interaction between a physician and her patient, one patient, sitting in front of one physician in her office. The resources available to that physician may differ based on policies, but the physician will still face one patient at a time.

Stacking the Deck

"You're looking at a cancer survivor," Nancy said repeatedly, during our first meeting in my office. Another physician had recently diagnosed her with a soft tissue sarcoma in the thigh that had already spread to the lungs. Due to an infection in the thigh mass, this other physician referred Nancy to me for urgent surgery to address that primary and infected site of the cancer so that she could safely pursue further chemotherapy.

I began our conversation after reviewing her history, imaging, and physical examination findings. "I don't mean to dampen your bright outlook or determination to get well, but you need to know a couple of things. I agree with your doctor that we need to deal first with the thigh, as it's currently preventing further treatment of the chest metastases. Nonetheless, you must know that the overall prognosis for patients with soft tissue sarcomas metastatic already when they present to medical attention is poor. The survival rate is low, about twenty percent at five years. Most of the patients who end up in that twenty percent surviving for five years will have one, two or three spots of metastatic disease only. In addition, they will usually experience a dramatic response of the tumor to chemo-therapy. You have more than three spots, and they have grown, rather than shrunk, during the first two cycles of chemotherapy."

"So I have no chance?"

"No. Don't misunderstand me. It isn't that you have no chance. You are young. This means that you can tolerate most chemo-therapy the medical oncologist can throw at your tumor. You are a mother of young children. This means that you will fight hard to live, which matters. Just because the first type of chemotherapy didn't appear to work doesn't mean the next one won't. The fact that we don't have a 'best' option chemotherapy for your type of sarcoma also means that we don't know that our 'second-best' option is really second. The oncologist may have simply guessed wrong the first time."

"So we cannot predict?"

"Exactly. We cannot predict. I can tell you that we know that less than five percent of patients in your exact situation will be alive in five years, but there are things we cannot know. Some physicians would call your case hopeless, but they would be wrong. It is hope-less if they say that 95 percent or even 98 percent is the same as 100 percent, but even 98 percent isn't 100. You must know that the chances are heavily stacked against you. They are not *impossibly* stacked against you."

How to make decisions in such slim-chance scenarios seriously challenges the accountants, bureaucrats, and administrators designing medical care systems. How many resources should we throw at conditions that are grossly unlikely to improve? One could easily argue that a medical system could safely ignore the entirety of my patient population without any blip in the wrong direction noticeable across the system's general population. Sarcomas are exceedingly rare as well as rather costly to manage, in terms of the resources they require.

However, only the number pushers far from the clinic room can really even consider such things. No one sitting in the room with Nancy could have told her that her desire to pursue a real --- albeit small --- chance for survival wouldn't receive the full support medicine could offer. Politicians and bureaucrats can haggle over the system constraints as much as they want. Nancy and I have enough trouble even if we unanimously determine to do all we can to aim for her best-case scenario.

Bean Counting

Another criticism leveled at health care in the United States is that we spend a large portion of the overall health expenditures for a person across his lifetime during the last few weeks of life.[5] I don't dispute this criticism. We can ascribe some of this problem to the fact that patients, their families, and physicians fail to face together the encroaching certainty of some patients' demise. Another large part of this over-spending of resources at the end of life derives from the difficulty in predicting the time of death. Even those desperate to live longer wouldn't ask that "everything" be done if they *knew* that the end encroached. Even physicians anxious to save their patients wouldn't recommend every possible intervention for a patient they *knew* would be dead in two weeks.

Most physicians know that they cannot predict the timing of death very well. This naturally results in some over-heroic attempts at delaying it in life's final hours. These heroic attempts also --- most definitely --- result in some dramatic saves from the jaws of impending death. Such saves may not make an impact that an epidemiologist can see. Such saves may cost more than they are worth to a bureaucrat or politician. But such saves might make all the difference in the world to an individual.

As reluctantly as physicians predict mortality, and as inaccurately as we predict when we dare, a desire to offer some level of expectation to emotionally charged situations prompts the occasional hazard of a guess at how much time a person has left. While we strictly avoid wagering money on such predictions, as insurance companies must, we often bet with currency much more dear. We often "spend" a portion of the time predicted to remain toward improving a later portion of that time, which the patient may or may not actually experience.

Many treatment decisions depend on some estimate of longevity. Should I fix the broken bone of a person dying from cancer? Will they die in two weeks or six months? No surgery I can offer will have helped appreciably by two weeks and might even have made them less comfortable for their final days. In contrast, most patients will not find my leaving them in bed or in a wheelchair for their final six months acceptable.

So how do we predict one patient at a time, when we must? To do this, physicians will occasionally use very crude prediction schemes similar to those used by life insurance actuaries, but not nearly as sophisticated. We call these disease-specific life prediction formulas nomograms. Usually derived from a series of patients with a given disease or condition, a nomogram will provide a calculator into which the physician inputs a few disease-specific variables. Such variables may be age, gender, and disease characteristics. The nomogram will then output a predicted percentage of patients expected to live so many months or so many years.

Physician utilization of many nomograms utterly befuddles me. We know they offer no more than wild guesses for some diseases. Do we think that adding mathematical calculations to our wild guesses improves them? I find such exercises amusing because physicians are so vigilant about the difference between individuals and populations on the side of gleaning principles, but forget this vigilance when *applying* principles. Physicians have a term for gleaning a principle from a single patient's experience. We call it anecdotal evidence.

As silly as it sounds, anecdotal evidence wields significant power. The human mind latches onto stories. Physicians criticize anecdotal evidence because we know how wildly an individual case may differ from any population-based reality. We forget that skepticism when we apply evidence gleaned from a population to a single patient in front of us. That single patient can still differ radically from the population-based expectation. Thus, when we predict using complicated nomogram formulas to spit out numbers, I have a hard time believing what those numbers can really mean to most patients.

We would not, I dare say, come anywhere close to the 8 percent profit margin that insurance companies regularly extract from their precise mortality predictions. Even when compared head-to-head with the frank guess of an experienced physician, many nomograms have fared worse in predicting patient longevity. The success of an experienced physician's best guess may have much to do with the impact of functional status on life expectancy in terminally ill patients.

Functional status is the level of livelihood, vigor, and capacity for general, independent self-care. It predicts longevity in cancer patients better than any other parameter or measure. Is it really a prediction? I think that it assesses more how much an individual has already begun the process of dying. While I may readily diagnose a patient as bound for death or even as being a certain distance along that decline toward death, I'll have much greater difficulty guessing the time course or pace of the remaining decline toward mortality itself.

Waiting the Odds

A few weeks ago, one of my chemotherapy-administering colleagues told me that one of our patients was dying. I had been away for a few days. She hoped to find me, thinking that the patient and her parents would appreciate a call from me. We had known the imminence of Lyla's death for many months, with slowly progressing metastatic sarcoma in her lungs. At the time she began her treatments as a 12-year-old, she already had metastasis. Unfortunately, chemotherapy had achieved little in the way of response.

Lyla's mother and I had spoken three months prior about what to expect along the winding way toward death. I had explained, quite honestly, that no one can really predict the timing with any precision.

"It could be as slow as a couple of years, or much faster, in terms of months. No matter what, a lot of tumor growth stands between our current confidence that her tumors are growing beyond our ability to stop them and the point at which they will fill enough of her lungs that she can even feel it. Frequently, a cancer will speed its pace, or gain momentum, as it grows, but if hers doesn't for some reason or another, it might still be many months."

"What do I do? Should I send her to school? Should I encourage her to keep up with her homework and piano practicing?" Lyla's mother had asked.

I had no good answers for her.

I learned from my colleague that the last few weeks had witnessed a clear gain in tumor momentum. Lyla's parents had brought her to the ER to evaluate shortness of breath during my week away. Imaging in the ER had shown that tumors had already replaced one whole lung as well as half the other lung. The ER team gave Lyla an oxygen tank. A hospice nurse scheduled visits to her home.

As a few days had passed since this discharge from the ER to die peacefully at home, my colleague sincerely worried that my call might come too late already. I checked with the service social worker to be sure that no calls had come from Lyla's parents announcing her passing, and then dialed their home number.

"Hello. Dr. Jones?" Lyla's father answered, recognizing my voice.

"Yes. How is she?"

"That's hard to say," he answered. "She is quite tired. She definitely needs the oxygen at times. Otherwise, though, she is still basically Lyla. I didn't expect her to last this long when we came home from the ER last week."

"Could I speak with her, by any chance?" I asked.

"She'd really love to talk to you, but she's napping right now. Do you want me to have her call you later this afternoon?"

"I am really calling to ask if it would it be okay if I came by tomorrow?"

"Are doctors allowed to make house calls these days?" he joked.

"I don't want to wear her out, as I know her energy and time are precious right now, but I would love the chance to stop by and see her for a few minutes."

"Of course, Doctor. Lyla would love to see you. We'd enjoy the visit too, if your schedule permits."

The next afternoon, Lyla's older brother let me in the front door.

"Dad is napping, and Mom decided to take a quick shower," he reported. "They weren't sure exactly when you would be here. They had a pretty rough night last night."

"I'm sorry to hear that," I offered. "If this is a bad time, I can call again at another."

I meant this sincerely but was happy when Lyla's brother shrugged off my protest.

"Lyla didn't have such a bad night, just Mom and Dad. She's in the other room playing a video game. She's been looking forward to your coming."

"Why did your parents have such a bad night?" I asked.

"Oh, my mom just seems to sit up most of the night watching Lyla sleep, waiting for something to happen."

"But nothing is happening."

"Not as far as we can tell, unless you count her beating me in this video game." This was clearly a jab at his little sister as we entered the room. "I'm not even letting her win these days."

Lyla grinned. She sat in her wheelchair. An oxygen mask hung lazily around her neck, its clear, thin hose twisting and winding down to the green tank beside her on the floor.

"My brother only got up to get the door because I was about to blast him anyway! He just used the doorbell as an excuse," Lyla said, and laughed. "How are you, Dr. Jones?"

"Fine. Thank you. How are you?"

"Oh, I feel okay. I have to keep this oxygen near, as I need it more often than not, but otherwise, I don't hurt or anything."

"She always says that her pain is at a 2 and that she doesn't want anything." Lyla's father had walked into the room behind me. He looked tired, his hair swept ungracefully to one side, doubtless from his just-ended nap. "Thank you so much for coming down, Dr. Jones."

"Thanks for allowing me to come."

"Pain hasn't been a big thing for us since Lyla came home from the hospital," Lyla's father continued. "They loaded us up with supplies of morphine and all, but she really hasn't needed anything. Kara asks her every couple of hours, but Lyla always seems to be okay. The hospice nurse checks in every afternoon to make sure our supply of pain meds is sufficient, but we really aren't using much."

"That's a good thing," I said.

"It is a good thing, but also a curious thing." Lyla's mother, looking fresher than her husband with her wet hair but otherwise just as sleep-deprived, had joined us. "Don't get me wrong. We're thrilled that Lyla isn't in pain. We're thrilled that Lyla is still strong. We just didn't expect our last week to go like this."

"Yup. The doctors at the hospital told me I was coming home to die," Lyla interjected rather matter-of-factly.

The visit continued pleasantly. We discussed a recent family vacation they had taken to Nashville. Lyla listed all the country music stars she had met there and how many of them had called her in the last week to check in on her. She played some of her favorite songs on the stereo for me. Eventually, she looked a bit tired, which reminded me to respect their family time. We said our goodbyes, which were not tearful. Lyla and I had talked about it before. I knew she had no fear of death. She had long ago accepted its approach.

Lyla's parents both walked me out to my car. Clearly, they wanted to talk more, out of earshot.

"What is happening?" Lyla's mother almost pleaded. "Don't misunderstand me. I love my daughter. I want to keep her here with us as long as possible, but this roller coaster is killing me. I almost feel like God is playing games with me, by making her look a little better every day."

"Well, she has good days and bad days," Lyla's father corrected. "Maybe I should say better days and worse days. But she seems a little stronger now than a week ago when we left the ER to come home for the end. As crazy as it sounds, it's hard to see her doing better, after we were prepared for her death. Kara and I can't sleep at night because we keep thinking that something must be about to happen, and we don't want to miss it."

"As her mother, I just can't stand the thought of Lyla feeling alone in her last moments."

"Functionally, that just means Kara stays up all night watching Lyla breathe," her father said.

Kara continued: "I have no idea how to manage this. If the end is near, we all want to focus all our attention on Lyla, spending time together and all. If she's doing better, do I try to start being a parent to my two boys as well? I'm swallowed by guilt every time I feel troubled that things aren't happening as we expected. I should be happy that we still have Lyla with us. I am happy. I just wish I knew what to expect each day."

I neither offered nor had any answers for Kara. She wasn't really asking me for answers. She knew that I didn't know. She and her husband knew that no one knows the future. They weren't at all unhappy with the team in the ER that had sent their daughter home to die. They knew it was happening, even if not in the prescribed few days.

Lyla's story is Lyla's story. No actuary's mortality experience is large enough or statistically robust enough to permit me or any other physician to predict the precise timing of Lyla's death. It will be her anecdote, only really told after it is complete.

Being Lucky and Good

Our inability to manage the uncertainty of death well is one of the great anxieties of modern culture. Some sections of society establish a legal framework for physician-assisted suicide, desperate to reduce the uncertainty of death as much as humanly possible.

Others fear directly interfering with the time of death, afraid that any influence they might bring to bear would be tantamount to playing God or even committing murder.

A friend of mine called me some months ago to discuss her husband's medical challenges. They have dealt with his chronic medical condition for most of their forty years of marriage. He was diagnosed with a progressive neuromuscular disease when their children, now grown, were very young. The progressive aspect has been in full force for more than a decade, binding him to a wheelchair and weakening even his capacity to invest effort in maintaining his strength.

So accustomed are they to ambulance visits to their home, trips to the ER, and one- to two-week hospital stays whenever his condition acutely worsens, that they easily take in stride these medical uncertainties. The prospect of his impending death doesn't fluster them. They have cherished the time already afforded them. They hope to enjoy more, but understand that his life's duration will be shortened. Their concern lately has been how to balance a desire to control the remaining quality of life without over-influencing the timing of death itself.

On this particular occasion, an episode had landed him in the ICU. Since admission to the ICU, his vital systems had returned to functional status. His consciousness hadn't. He wasn't in a coma. He wasn't overmedicated into a sleepy stupor. He just was less than fully awake and aware most of the time. He had experienced lucid moments. He had recognized his wife a few times. He had once acknowledged the presence of two of his children. He was not, at the present, acknowledging the presence of food when it was placed in front of him.

The care team had placed a feeding tube through one of his nostrils. They asked his wife to decide whether or not they should surgically place a more permanent feeding tube through the stomach wall to sustain him. She asked me to review her thinking with her, as a friend.

"I'm not afraid of his dying. I know that he isn't afraid of his dying. We got over that, years ago. I just don't want to. . . well. . . cause it."

"You don't want to play God," I clarified.

"Absolutely," she agreed.

"I have good news for you, then. In none of the options you are considering *can* you play God. You can't determine when your husband will die, unless you poison him or overdose some dangerous medication, or do him a physical harm in some way that you are far from considering."

I continued, "You are trying to maintain his quality of life. You and he have agreed to the limits of intervention when the end of his life is approaching."

"But how do I know that *now* is when that end is approaching?" she interrupted.

"To some extent it has been approaching for a long time, hasn't it?" I asked.

"But when is it imminent enough to prompt a change in decisions?"

"Ah. That's much more difficult to say. You no doubt know whether or not it's imminent much better than I can. You probably know better than his physicians."

"That doesn't help, though," she noted.

"You just have to understand that no one can know exactly when death is coming. If we could, it might make all of our decisions easier. Or would it?"

"What do you mean?" she asked.

"Okay, my comment may not be fair. You asked when death will be imminent enough to change your decisions. I'm not sure that the imminence of death *should* change your decisions, beyond the fact that you already know that he has a disease that will take him sooner than later. I would argue that not knowing exactly when it will take him actually helps your decisions. It is more freeing than binding. Go through this line of thought with me for a minute. First, you're trying to manage your husband's comfort while awaiting the uncertain timing of death. Second, you are determined not to play God and decide the timing of his death."

"Right."

"Well, the glorious thing is that any intervention you request or deny to nudge his comfort situation is just as uncertain in its effects on the timing of death as the timing of death is uncertain in and of itself."

"Meaning that the power I wield in the decisions I am considering is much less than I worry it might be," she concluded.

"Exactly," I agreed. "This doesn't make these decisions go away, but it can remove from them some of the anxiety about playing God."

"But if we don't put in a permanent feeding tube, the nose tube will almost certainly get infected or clogged or have some other problem."

"*Almost* certainly. That 'almost' is really important. No intervention or lack thereof is sure to have the desired benefits or undesired side effects. Neither is the necessity of any intervention as clear as you might think. You have no idea if he'll wake up tomorrow with a big appetite and no longer need any tube. You have no idea if he'll die peacefully in his sleep tonight, making this whole consideration moot.

"Even if you removed the feeding tube that is in him, you wouldn't be killing your husband. You simply don't know what the removal of that intervention would do to him."

"So nothing matters?"

"Your decisions matter, but you can't be sure how any intervention will matter with regard to the length of his life. Make your decisions independent from his prognosis as best you can. Worry about comfort measures first, life-prolonging measures second."

I have no idea if my thoughts helped my friend or not. Her husband recovered some strength over the days following our conversation. He actually made it home from the hospital a couple of weeks later. He was home for less than a month, this time with a shared decision they both made to refuse any more ambulance trips to the ER. When he died, both he and his wife were at peace with their decision.

A prominent businessman in our community also recently died. His life demonstrated Midas' golden touch. Although I know his life story wasn't free from challenges, he struck me as one who could manage things well. He managed life and family well; he managed a complex business conglomerate including a number of companies well; he even managed to die well. As it became clear to him and his physicians that his active and progressive medical problems were poised to take his life, he went home from the hospital, gathered all of his children and grandchildren around him, and had nearly a week with them, saying goodbyes, giving final advice, enjoying family time together before his passing.

The time might have been too short to manage that special family time together. It might have been long and drawn out, prompting family members to be too long away from their other responsibilities as they waited with him for weeks. It turned out just about right. Some would say he was lucky. He would say he was blessed. Either way, for the dying part itself, he wasn't in control. He could only receive, not necessarily improve, his mortality experience.

Starting Your Conversation. . . .

Paying the Bills

Principle: One can make predictions for a population based on observations of that population over time. Such predictions don't easily apply to one member of the population at a time.
Ask your physician: What have you observed in other patients you have seen with my condition?

Gambling

Principle: Actuaries in the life insurance industry observe and apply death statistics from large populations to make predictions very accurately for large populations. They call the deaths for which their company pays out their mortality experience.
Ask your physician: How many successes and failures have you personally witnessed among patients with my condition?

Working Population

Principle: Health systems can variably focus on individuals or the entire population, the former limiting its ability to control health variables that matter from a bird's-eye view, the latter limiting its ability to offer maximal flexibility to individuals and their individual physicians.
Ask your physician: Does my insurance change the options that you and I can consider and pursue at this point?

Stacking the Deck

Principle: We pursue some very slim chances for some very motivated patients because we have no way of measuring possibilities, only probabilities. For these patients, uncertainty is the only source of hope.
Ask your physician: Would other physicians in your field agree with you that my chances are reasonable to pursue?

Bean Counting

Principle: When we must, physicians make predictions based on small populations of patients who have a diagnosis in common, then dangerously apply it to one patient at a time.

Ask your physician: On how many patients is your best guess based?

Waiting the Odds

Principle: Physician predictions aim at the average, but patients can experience the extremes.

Ask your physician: What is the range of possible outcomes for my condition so that I can prepare for the extremes of that range, as well as the average?

Being Lucky and Good

Principle: Sometimes we make our best decisions as we near the end of life if we ignore survival entirely in the moment of decision.

Ask your physician: If I am not worried about length of life, how will this treatment influence my experience of whatever life remains?

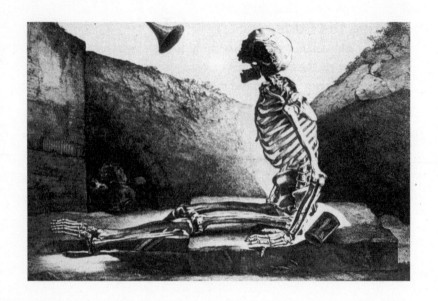

WILL IT TAKE AN ACT OF CONGRESS?

Afraid to Say

"Kevin, I won't be able to have lunch with you as planned. I'll be at the hospital for some tests."

My former English literature professor and I often met for lunch during my weekend trips back to Boston during my first year of medical school in Baltimore. This particular teacher and I had established a friendship during a few classes and a one-on-one tutorial we had shared during my college years. He had retired as I had graduated. He and his wife still lived near campus.

"My doctor ordered some initial tests as he planned to start me on a cholesterol pill," he continued. "When he saw those results, he told me he was interested in my liver. I told him that I wanted to have the most boring liver he had ever come across!"

My friend's liver did prove interesting to his physician, unfortunately. A month later, anticipating another visit to Boston, I had planned lunch with him.

Our telephone call planning our meeting ended with this: "And Kevin, I want to ask you some questions when you come. They found some spots in my liver, apparently from my pancreas."

Over lunch a few days later, I learned that a biopsy of the liver masses had identified metastatic pancreatic cancer.

"They don't see any mass in the pancreas itself," he explained, "but they seem certain that it is where the spots came from. They had me meet an oncologist who wants to start chemotherapy."

I wasn't far along in medical school but knew enough to know that pancreatic cancer is an extremely deadly disease even when not already metastatic to the liver. I also knew how to find more information.

My search for articles found no cases of long-term survival reported from metastatic pancreatic cancer treated with any regimen. It became obvious to me that my friend's oncologist planned chemotherapy of palliative (intended to minimize symptoms) rather than curative intent.

Our remaining lunches relocated from restaurants to the living room in his house. We had very few of these before a call came from his son, sharing the news that my friend had passed. "My mom asked me to call you. She said my dad wanted you to know when it happened."

From the time he learned of his diagnosis, my professor and I both knew what the final outcome would be. Doubtless, his oncologist knew as well.

"Why hasn't he told me that?" my friend asked me at one point.

As much as he sensed the end coming, he insisted that his oncologist had never mentioned that the chemotherapies they were trying were never even intended to cure, only to quiet symptoms. He rationalized that all conversations with his oncologist were brief and that they never discussed much of anything else in detail either, but this detail bothered him.

"Why won't he say it?" he asked me. "It's clear to me that I am dying. I have less energy every week. My belly is so full of fluid I can hardly stand from this chair."

Eventually, my professor had asked for no more chemo, as it nauseated him and didn't seem to be working. The oncologist had quickly finished that visit and didn't schedule any more appointments.

My friend was certainly grieving and may not have caught the detail about palliative intent in his first meeting with the oncologist. I know that many of my own patients miss details of our conversations when trying to process volumes of emotionally charged information.

I still don't understand how the oncologist never directly discussed the fact that my friend was dying. Here was a Harvard English professor, really a professional communicator, a deft writer and skilled lecturer; surely, he could understand any message, however painful.

His impending death was in no way uncertain. Perhaps the exact timing was yet to be experienced, but he wasn't going to survive for long. He lasted about nine months beyond his diagnosis, actually some weeks longer than typical for metastatic pancreatic carcinoma.

Did the oncologist fear his patient could not handle the finality of such a prognosis? Does this follow the same problem we saw in full disclosure of uncertainty itself? Do physicians fear that patients will seek another physician if they paint an insufficiently rosy picture of the expected outcomes?

Totally Telling

Physicians don't have or don't deftly execute a number of important conversations with their patients. Apparent from my professor's experience, physicians sometimes invest lackluster effort in speaking honestly with their patients about death. Physicians fail in other conversations about prognosis in spite of our best efforts. We do a very poor job of explaining what to expect in potential complications or even anticipated side effects from treatments we plan.

Nerve injuries are one example in my field. These are, thankfully, rare. They might complicate any limb surgery though. Positioning alone can cause nerves to stop working during surgery. Most surgeons mention nerve injury during a discussion of surgical risks. The lawyers tell us we must. Most surgeons then quickly point out that nerves are almost never accidentally severed in the course of the operation. They may then add the caveat that nerves don't need to be severed to stop working. Pressure from retraction, positioning, or changes in limb alignment all can cause nerve palsies.

Surgeons rarely predict that these nerve palsies from stretch- or pressure-damage incidents will be devastating. Yes, many recover with time, but that time might be months or even years. Some never recover. While a nerve isn't functioning, some surgeons will note, muscle control and skin sensation provided by the nerve will not work properly. Very few surgeons emphasize the worst expected part of severe nerve palsies, the nerve pain that can plague the patient with feelings of boiling water poured down the limb without warning.

Most surgeons shudder even to think of these worst-case scenarios, let alone discuss them with patients. They are exceedingly rare, but they are not "never" events. Should such prognoses be dwelt on? Probably not, but they lurk out there. Perhaps surgeons shouldn't dwell on them because, even if explained, what good would it do? How many patients who ultimately experience such a complication will have been truly prepared to experience it from the conversation? None. Even if not legally a surprise, this will be an experiential surprise to everyone who endures these rare worst-case scenarios.

I am confident of this surprise phenomenon because there are adverse outcomes or side effects that arise in a completely *anticipated* fashion that aren't nearly as dramatic as nerve palsies and yet still surprise patients. The experience of healing a split thickness skin graft is one such surprising experience.

I go to great lengths explaining to patients who will have a split-thickness skin graft as a part of an upcoming surgery that it will positively disgust them while it is healing. I explain that it will weep and ooze, then get crusty and scabbed, all of this persisting over a number of weeks. I even tell them to expect to be surprised by how gross it will look to them.

Without fail, even with grins on their faces as they remember aloud our pre-operative conversation, each one will have some moment in a follow-up setting in which I tell her that her skin graft looks great and appears exactly as it should appear and she responds with, "Really? Are you sure there isn't something wrong?"

There are some experiences for which conversations cannot entirely prepare a person.

I think of one young man from whose chest wall and ribs I planned to remove a tumor. I explained that it would require a chest tube, which would be very uncomfortable.

"What do you mean?" he asked.

"Well, for the three to four days that this chest tube will stay in," I explained, "every cough and even every breath will stab you with pain. The anesthesiologist may be able to numb up a rib or two with an injection, but if that fails, you will basically hate my guts with every breath you take, especially when you laugh or cough."

I'll never forget my conversation with him two days after his surgery. The rib nerve blocks from anesthesia hadn't worked well. He was having some difficulty with the pain.

"I had no idea it was going to hurt this badly!" he sputtered in shallow breaths, trying to avoid breathing deeply and exacerbating the pain.

"Do you hate me right now?" I asked.

"No. You totally told me this would happen. I just didn't believe you."

Was I vindicated? Yes, of course. Had I effectively prepared him for what was coming? No. I have to ask, how could I?

Some argue that non-physicians with more time to talk, or movies or photos can better educate patients for what they are about to --- or may be about to --- experience. This might be true. I spend lots of time with my patients, followed by a nurse who spends even more. But I am convinced that some ends known from the beginning will always be difficult to communicate at the beginning to patients who will experience them in the end.

Even certainties become uncertain when we try to communicate them to another person.

Sweating the Small Stuff

One of the most difficult experiences for which I must occasionally prepare patients is the experience of uncertainty itself. I recently failed at just such a communication with a friend who became a patient.

Many of my patients become my friends, but the opposite rarely occurs for me. Sure, I will suture minor lacerations, set and cast a few children's fractures, and do the occasional Boy Scout physical for neighbors, but those in my modest social acquaintance don't develop the one-in-a-million-rare cancer diagnoses in whose care I specialize at a rate sufficient to fill my clinics.

They probably develop these rare cancers at the same rate as all the people with whom I have not interacted socially, but I don't have a million friends! I will often note to friends that they don't want to have the diagnoses that land them in my clinic.

When my friend became a cancer patient, he was my patient for only a brief interlude; he remains my friend. At a routine check-up with his primary care physician, Luke had undergone biopsy of a skin lesion on his shoulder. When the physician notified him of a diagnosis of melanoma, Luke called me to learn whom he should see at my cancer center for definitive management.

I arranged for him to see two specialists, one to surgically remove the melanoma from his shoulder skin, the second to initiate a surveillance program to track any other moles. Luke met with both of these excellent physicians, had the melanoma removed, and initiated the surveillance program with a baseline examination and photographs to map any existing moles. The pathologist ultimately judged his melanoma to be low-risk overall. Luke heard that he could expect a 90- to 95-percent survival rate. He would follow-up for continued surveillance in 6 months unless he or his wife noticed any moles visibly changing before then.

When his wife raised concern a month later about two additional moles on his back, she called the clinic. The melanoma surveillance expert could not see Luke until a month later, but would biopsy the lesions at that time. Still not emotionally settled about his recently positive biopsy and the 5- to 10-percent chance of death it portended for him, Luke panicked a little at this scheduling.

My friend therefore became my patient, in that I would perform the biopsies and send the results to the melanoma experts.

The pathologist called one of the skin spots a pre-cancerous lesion, possibly on its way toward melanoma. She recommended slightly wider excision. After performing this second minor surgery, Luke and I discussed his results again as well as the overall picture.

"How do I keep from going crazy about every mole I have on my body?" he asked.

"You've hired the best guy I know to watch these for you. Do your best to let him worry about them. That's his job, and he's good at it."

"But even one of these was pre-cancerous already."

"Yes, but it is also the one he told you to watch most closely," I countered.

"A month from now, it might have already become full-blown melanoma.

"I doubt that very much. I intervened to address emotional urgency, not medical urgency," I explained.

"I know. I know. I just couldn't even see it myself, which worried me more. I can't yet get over the fact that the one that was melanoma might even be in me, lurking somewhere."

"The chances that it isn't are overwhelming though," I reminded him.

"Still, 5- to 10-percent of the time it will show up somewhere else in a lymph node or worse and end up killing me."

"Your chances of distant relapse are likely much lower than that, all things considered. However, forget the number; what can you do about it?" I asked.

"What do you mean?"

"What can you do about the fact that some small risk floats out there that your original melanoma will come back? What can you possibly do about it? Nothing. Even worrying about it won't make you better at picking it up or anything else in this case. Please, worry about the fact that you can get a second melanoma. Worry about it *just enough* to wear sun block and protect your skin when you are out. Worry about it *enough* to show up for your surveillance appointments in the melanoma clinic. Worrying beyond that accomplishes nothing for you. It's good that you know that there is a chance that it can come back so that you make wise decisions with your time and resources. Wallowing in that uncertainty will not help you though."

Luke hadn't yet settled into his on-going and unalterable state of uncertainty. I expect that he'll grow a bit more comfortable in that experience with time. No conversation could have hoped to prepare him for it. I doubt that our conversation even helped him get through the experience of the ongoing uncertainty after he arrived in the midst of it. As much as I have focused on honest communication as the answer to uncertainty throughout this book, even honesty cannot erase the experience of uncertainty.

Drained

I don't think that Charlie had any idea when he came to the ER that night that he had a serious problem. He sought medical attention at 11 PM because he had finished his shift at the factory at ten. For two weeks, he'd noticed some mild shortness of breath whenever he lay down. He knew he smoked too much and planned, as so many do, to quit sometime soon. He guessed that his shortness of breath had something to do with his smoking; he felt he needed to get it checked. He knew he was too young at 52 and too healthy otherwise to have such trouble breathing.

The internal medicine team I was rotating with as a medical student admitted Charlie to the hospital when we found that a collection of fluid had collapsed his lung on one side. We watched him closely overnight, but no significant new problems developed. His breathing eased slightly after receiving some emphysema medications. His wife joined him in the hospital after she got their two high-school-aged children off to school the next morning. We performed a thoracentesis, or needle drainage of the fluid, which improved his symptoms dramatically. He also had a CT scan later in the morning, which showed one large and a few smaller masses in the lungs, consistent with a lung carcinoma.

We scheduled a pulmonologist to biopsy one of the lesions using a scope the next day, but little doubt remained in the diagnosis. He asked us if we could meet and speak with his teenage kids if they came to the hospital after school that day. Of course, we agreed to do so. As the medical student assigned to his case from our service, I was invited to attend.

The family meeting proceeded uneventfully. Charlie's wife asked how fast things might progress if this turned out to be the expected lung cancer. We explained that metastatic lung cancers can be rapid in their progress, leaving their victims only a few months to settle affairs and say goodbyes. We explained that once the biopsy achieved a tissue diagnosis we would refer him to the oncology team to plan chemotherapy, even if only palliative. He would stay in the hospital overnight but might even go home after the biopsy the following morning. He already felt so much better with the fluid drained and the lung re-inflated.

I left the hospital that night somewhat energized by having witnessed such a discussion. Obviously, Charlie's situation shocked his family and still dripped with uncertainty, but I had enjoyed watching the gently orchestrated discussion unfold. I felt the attending physician had executed his role well. What was known was told. What wasn't yet known was acknowledged. Comfort was given.

Having been on admitting call the night before when Charlie came in, this night, our team was off. Our patients were to be covered by a resident from another team.

Arriving the next morning, I checked first in Charlie's room before heading to our workroom. The lights were out, the bed empty and freshly made. Assuming that nursing staff must have switched his room, I continued on to our team's workroom. There, a chalkboard bore a list of our patients, the residents and medical students assigned to each, and their room numbers.

An eraser smear replaced Charlie's name on our list. As none of our team's residents was in yet, I wandered to the other team's room, looking for someone with any answers. A resident in wrinkled scrubs and a white coat sat, poring over notes, alone. She had a sufficiently disheveled look to declare unequivocally that she had been the one on-call overnight.

"What happened to Mr. Mattson?" I asked.

"Oh!" She was startled by my interruption of her work. "He gave me a terrible night. He awoke with breathing trouble in the middle of the night. You guys hadn't changed him from full code status." This is the designation in the medical record that physicians should do "everything" to keep a patient alive. Specifically, some patients with terminal conditions will ask not to have CPR, transfer to an ICU, or intubation and mechanical breathing performed if their condition deteriorates.

She continued: "I called his wife to see if she wanted me to tube him or not. Since he's dying anyway, she opted against it. He died before she got here. What a mountain of paperwork! Then they didn't come get his body until 4 AM. As if I didn't have enough to worry about with the rest of my patients who were still alive. Sad story, too! He is awfully young to die of lung CA. Can you let your resident and attending know what happened when they get here? I still have a lot to do to get my other patients ready for our rounds."

"Sure. . . . Will he have an autopsy?"

"Are you crazy? Do you think I was going to bring that up? The family was already in shock. They didn't need that as an additional stress." She refocused her attention on the papers in front of her. "Just be sure to explain to your attending what happened."

Our conversation had clearly come to an end, so I walked back to my own team's workroom. Not knowing the resident personally, I happily attributed her abrupt, callous manner to the usual post-call punchiness. The rest of the botching of Charlie's death was our fault. Not that he died. We clearly had no power to predict or long-prohibit that. We failed in that we postponed uncomfortable conversations until the moment of duress.

We had no way of guessing that Charlie would decline so rapidly. We'll never know exactly what did it. He likely developed something only tangentially related to the tumor in his chest. Without anticipating its sudden timing, we felt we had covered quite a lot in the family meeting only hours before Charlie's death.

Quite a lot was not, explicitly, quite enough.

The on-call resident, unknown to the family and only vaguely acquainted with the details of Charlie's situation from her sign-out sheet, couldn't have done better. She spent her one admissible shock conversation with Mrs. Mattson to cover the issue of CPR and intubation in the setting of likely terminal cancer. She couldn't easily have also asked, "By the way, since this is so unexpected, can we have an autopsy performed to be sure we have the right diagnosis?"

Even though we failed to add code status to our discussion with the patient, he might have discussed such matters with his wife prior to her moment of decision --- but he probably had not. Far too few people actually have such conversations when they should, when they are well and in no apparent immediate danger of imminent death.

All of us will die at some point. This is certain. Some of us will go out with a sudden bang in a massive trauma or stroke, heart attack or pulmonary embolism, leaving no decisions for our loved ones to make for us. Most, though, will not go out suddenly and with our wits about us. Telling someone how we feel about end-of-life issues and decision-making liberates our loved ones from the pain of making those decisions for us. Those tough decisions can agonize a person less if he senses that he is simply enacting goals agreed upon in conversation weeks, months or years earlier.

Bad-tasting Medicine

Since that time, I have a few times been in the shoes of the resident, arranging last-minute discussions with family members as important decisions approached regarding the level of care desired for a critically ill patient. Certainly, the medical assessment of the patient's prognosis figures into these discussions, but much more emotional are the family members' grasping attempts to guess what the patient would have wanted. Sometimes the answer is obvious and its determination awaits only the arrival of some distant family member to support emotionally the one with decision-making power.

Rarely, family members will disagree. When they do, family drama escalates. Not only will discussion long before the moment prevent some of these emotional fiascos, it can enable decision-making in real time. Discussion ahead of time can powerfully change the very decisions that need to be made. It can preempt the creation of a situation in which a family must choose whether or not to remove interventions.

One decides more easily *not to begin* a life-prolonging intervention than *not to continue* a life-prolonging intervention after successful initiation. Prior to starting the intervention, one cannot predict its success in prolonging even technical life. If a spouse decides not to pursue connection to a breathing machine for her husband, she does so before knowing whether the breathing machine would even work to sustain his body. This uncertainty comforts any decision not to begin an intervention. Once applied and successful --- at least temporarily --- the intervention's success at least appears more certain, rendering its potential removal less emotionally comfortable.

We are all familiar with the Terri Schiavo case and its many legal and ultimately legislative battles.[1] As we know from news sources and media outlets, Terri Schiavo's heart stopped in her home. Although attended to by emergency responders, whose CPR successfully restored circulation, the duration of stalled circulation created a severe brain injury.

Terri persisted in a coma for months, and then eventually emerged into what is termed a "persistent vegetative state." By report, her husband, still hopeful for recovery, attempted a number of measures to reinvigorate brain function. These included an electric brain stimulator and many diverting excursions to expose her to external environmental stimulation. None of these interventions changed her mental status appreciably.

Perhaps from a rising hopelessness, perhaps from devious goals of inheriting his wife's money (the latter ascribed to him by her parents), Terri's husband then began to question the wisdom in keeping Terri alive in this vegetative state.

Apparently, three years following the brain injury, Terri's husband requested a do-not-resuscitate order (the opposite of the full-code status that remained in Charlie's case, discussed previously) in the setting of a urinary tract infection, which she had contracted. Terri's condition never deteriorated badly enough to need CPR during the days or weeks in which this do-not-resuscitate order was on the books. Eventually, her husband retracted the do-not-resuscitate order, returning Terri to full-code status.

Purportedly, he had requested the order having reasoned that she had no meaningful hope for recovery. He sought some life-saving intervention that he could avoid initiating, rather than having to withdraw something that was already working. His decision was based on a poor prognosis. I can only assume that his decision to undo that do-not-resuscitate order arose from a different opinion regarding the prognosis.

Five years later, Terri's husband petitioned the court to have her feeding tube removed. The fact that he petitioned the court suggests that legal battles were already under way at this point, but the legal details aren't critical to our discussion. Terri's parents opposed this action. The court appointed a guardian to consider Terri's best interests. The guardian's report and the decisions that followed are frankly fascinating to me in their twisted reasoning.

After discussing her case with many physicians involved in Terri's care, the guardian concluded that she met the legal definition of a persistent vegetative state and that there was no possibility of improvement. However, the guardian also suspected that Terri's husband was motivated by conflicting interests, that he hoped to inherit her remaining estate. This conflict of interest also implicated her parents, who stood to become heirs-at-law if they won their legal battle of guardianship. Due to these complicating conflicts of interest, the guardian deemed this prognosis of no possibility of improvement irrelevant and denied feeding tube removal.

Two years later, nearly a decade from her original brain injury, a trial determined again that she was in a persistent vegetative state and that she had made oral declarations to friends prior to her incident that she wouldn't want a feeding tube in such a situation. Her parents maintained that as a devout Catholic, she would never have requested death by starvation.

After her parents mounted another challenge to guardianship that the court denied, a new date was set for tube removal a few months later. When the tube was removed, Terri's parents filed a civil suit of perjury against her husband. This brought the case to a new court that demanded the tube be reinserted until the new case was settled. Despite a couple of suits by her husband, the tube was reinserted five days after removal.

The next round of appeals focused on challenging the diagnosis and prognosis itself. No one needs to look further than this hearing to see blatant prognostic uncertainty. Of the five physicians appointed to review the case, four were neurologists and one a radiologist. They reviewed a new CT scan showing severe brain atrophy (sickly thinning), an electroencephalogram (EEG) showing no electrically measurable brain activity, and a 6-hour video of Terri. The two physicians added to the panel by Terri's parents reported that she was "minimally conscious" as opposed to "persistently vegetative" in mental state. The court ruled otherwise and that the tube should come out.

Terri's parents went further to post 6 minutes from the 6-hour video on the web; to them, the clips suggested meaningful movement on Terri's part. They attempted re-litigation of the entire case by producing new witnesses of Terri's care during a period seven years prior. When the courts silenced this attempt, the parents lobbied the Florida state legislature. It passed a law giving the governor the power to intervene, which he did, having the tube reinserted after this second court-ordered removal. The District and then the Supreme Court of Florida then ruled this governor-enabling legislation unconstitutional.

As publicity for the case expanded, Terri's parents brought a petition signed by a number of physicians, demanding a functional MRI and swallowing therapy with VitalStim. The judge ruled that these attempts were experimental and that the feeding tube should be removed.

A U.S. congressional hearing was then called, which resulted in the passage of a law that transferred the case to Federal courts from the State. Despite this bipartisan political flourish, Federal courts also denied Terri's parents' appeals. Notwithstanding a near showdown between state and local law enforcement, the feeding tube was removed, and Terri expired six days later.

I don't broach this horrific case with the suggestion that I know what *ought* to have happened. An argument for or against maintenance of the feeding tube could easily be made. At some points in the many hearings and rulings, Terri's parents actually argued that for religious reasons, regardless of the expected prognosis, they didn't want the euthanasia that they saw in tube removal to take place. But through most of the case this idealistic moral high ground can't be claimed by either party.

Mostly, this case came down to prognosis. What was the chance of return to cognitive function from Terri's persistent vegetative state, and how was that chance determined? The fact that licensed, presumably honest physicians came down on both sides of the debate exposes the uncertainty inherent in such predictions.

The Terri Schiavo case employed a broad array of technology to define, or really diagnose, her mental status. So, in some way, we have come full circle, back to uncertainty in diagnosis.

CT scans and MRIs can offer only the shapes and sizes of different parts of the brain. In terms of diagnosis, it is generally agreed that when many brain cells die, the brain cortex shrinks dramatically and is termed atrophic. EEG and functional MRI both try to represent not shapes as much as activity in the neural circuits of the brain, the former by subtle electrical charges traveling through nerves, the latter by uptake of a specific signal-enhancing molecule. Each technology has advantages and disadvantages, as well as uncertainty intrinsic to its interpretation.

As is common to many stories reviewed in this book, the final word came from a pathologist, this time in an autopsy setting, who noted that the entire cortex of Terri's brain was shriveled and dead. Even of this diagnosis --- you know now --- one can ask, what does it mean? Well, that is, unfortunately, uncertain.

Only one thing is certain to me from Terri Schiavo's story. Whatever the outcome, I don't want my end-of-life medical decisions made via YouTube blog responses, radio and television pundits, courts or the United States Congress.

Communicating with your spouse and family about your wishes on these issues is absolutely critical. More and more people these days are filing living wills and medical powers of attorney; this is a good trend. These documents may be very helpful if family melodrama erupts as it did for the Schiavos. However, the documents are not the most important piece. Most important are the conversations you have with your loved ones. As uncomfortable as such conversations may be to have now, not having had them will be even more uncomfortable when the time for conversations has passed, but the need for their application is present.

April 15th

Some say that the only two things certain in life are death and taxes. You can only predict the timing of the latter with precision.

On the computer monitor in front of me in the ICU bay, I watched Gerald dying from the hall outside his room. I was the intern responsible for his care.

His two adult children had arrived to say goodbye and support his wife, their mother. She had decided not to pursue resuscitation when things had gone badly with his heart after a motor vehicle accident. Gerald had served in the Second World War, farmed corn and beans on a large acreage in northeast Iowa and raised two happy and successful children, who had provided grandchildren and even a great-grandchild to him and his beloved wife of more than 50 years.

No one could have expected that the other driver coming toward his tractor had fallen asleep in the early morning hours, or that when Gerald was thrown from the tractor he would severely bruise the heart muscle. From the combination of his age and the severity of his chest injury, one could expect --- even on arrival at the hospital --- that things wouldn't go well.

As the accident happened very near their farm home, Gerald's wife had followed the ambulance in her car. She notified the physician team of her husband's wishes not to have drastic measures taken to prolong life dependent on machines. She hoped that we could support him long enough for their children to arrive.

As his heartbeats had begun to spread out in time, Gerald's wife and I both noticed a change in his countenance. Was it skin color? Was it reduced muscle tone? Was it his spirit leaving his dying body? Neither of us knew, but the room was peaceful and quiet.

When his son and daughter arrived, a few minutes after that change in countenance, I left them alone, with the lights turned down. After nearly an hour, his breathing had stopped, but the heart kept beating, more slowly, more slowly. Eventually, the weak EKG pulses were more than a minute apart. Then they were gone. A few minutes later, Gerald's son opened the door and motioned to me.

"I think Dad's passed."

"Yes, I think he has."

I entered the room, checked for a pulse as a perfunctory examination, and then quietly left them. After a few more minutes in the room, the three left. The son had brought the number of their local mortician. He had called the mortuary while on the way to the hospital. The mortician would send his team to get the body. The whole event could not have gone more smoothly. Gerald had passed peacefully.

I set about my responsibility of death paperwork before returning to my other patients in the surgical intensive care unit. That paperwork provided a variety of boxes to fill in the detailed cause, time and location of death. "Where" was easy enough and even "cause," heart failure secondary to cardiac contusion secondary to motor vehicle accident, but "when?"

I knew the specific hour and minute when I had "pronounced" him dead, which certainly sufficed for the paperwork. The exact minute really didn't matter a great deal for this peaceful passing, happily devoid of melodrama. But when had Gerald actually died? When his countenance changed? When brain activity stopped? When he stopped breathing? The moment immediately after the last heartbeat? Or the moment two minutes later when it became apparent that the next beat wasn't actually coming? I have no idea.

The uncertainty of death goes far beyond the inability to *predict* its timing. It is often rather difficult to be sure even when it has arrived.

Death's arrival is so uncertain that a physician must declare or pronounce it. As if we really know. We are reasonably skilled at identifying the absence of signs of life or making the diagnosis of death; but when, between the presence of signs of life and their declared or pronounced absence they actually depart is completely unknown.

Closing Time

That same year in which I witnessed Gerald's heartbeats pass to silence, I heard a story. I cannot confirm its veracity. It smacks of medical lore and legend more than reality, but it isn't strictly impossible. I tell it because it perfectly illustrates my point of the difficulty of pronouncing the arrival of death.

The story goes that a prominent cardiac surgeon at a nationally prominent university medical center was performing open-heart surgery with his fellow-in-training. After restoring blood supply to the heart muscle through coronary artery bypasses, they had difficulty getting the heart started again so that the patient could be disconnected from the heart-lung machine. The heart muscle would start to squeeze for a minute or so, then seize up again.

Once it started for long enough to get the patient disconnected from the heart-lung machine and even close up the chest wound, but then stopped again. CPR had commenced with effects similar to the surgeon's efforts with the chest open: start pumping again for a few minutes, then stop.

Finally, when the heart failed to start after a longer duration of CPR, the faculty surgeon stepped back from the table, mimed a dusting motion of his gloved hands and proclaimed, "He's dead. We are the best. We have done our best. The heart isn't working. He's dead. John, don't forget to talk to the family; they knew this might be coming." He then walked out of the operating room.

But John persisted in CPR. After another 15 or 20 minutes of starting, then stopping again, the heart began to beat and maintained a rhythm. The patient was transferred to the cardiac surgical intensive care unit and actually did well overnight. By mid-morning the next day, the ICU nurse paged the faculty surgeon. "I just wanted to know when you are planning on rounding today, so I can let the family know when to expect you. Mr. Akins is doing really well."

Before going to the ICU, the faculty surgeon paged John, his fellow, for a teaching moment. "John?"

"Yes, sir?" John answered.

"The nurse just called me to tell me that Mr. Akins is alive and that his family is waiting for me."

"I'm sorry, sir," John apologized. "I was pulled to help with another emergency and forgot to call you to let you know that we finally got his heart going again."

"John. . . ."

"Yes, sir?"

"The next time I tell you my patient is dead, you leave him dead!"

Starting Your Conversation. . . .

Afraid to Say

Principle: Just as physicians struggle to tell what they don't know, they may also struggle to admit what they know that isn't pleasant.

Ask your physician: What are your goals for this treatment? May I share my goals with you?

Totally Telling

Principle: Physicians also struggle to prepare patients for expected but unfavorable outcomes.

Ask your physician: What has surprised patients most as they experience these treatments or this disease course?

Sweating the Small Stuff

Principle: One singularly difficult experience for which to prepare through conversation is the experience of on-going uncertainty after active treatments are complete.

Ask your physician: How much of my present uncertainty will remain after treatment?

Drained

Principle: There is no time like the present to discuss what will happen if a patient loses the capacity to make decisions for herself.

Ask your physician: What should we discuss now that we might not be able to discuss if my condition worsens more rapidly than expected?

Bad-tasting Medicine

Principle: As difficult as they are, conversations between each of us and our loved ones to help them understand how we feel about end-of-life issues are critical to have before the hour of need.

Ask your physician: Do you know whom to contact if I become incapable of making decisions for myself?

Ask your family or at least your next-of-kin: Do you know how I feel about my own end-of-life?

April 15th

Principle: Even confirming the arrival of death can be difficult.

Ask your physician: (Especially if you hope to be an organ donor) How will you determine when I have died?

Closing Time

Principle: The uncertainty of death's arrival means that a physician ultimately decides that someone has died and stops trying to reverse this state.

Ask your physician: When/how will we decide to stop trying?

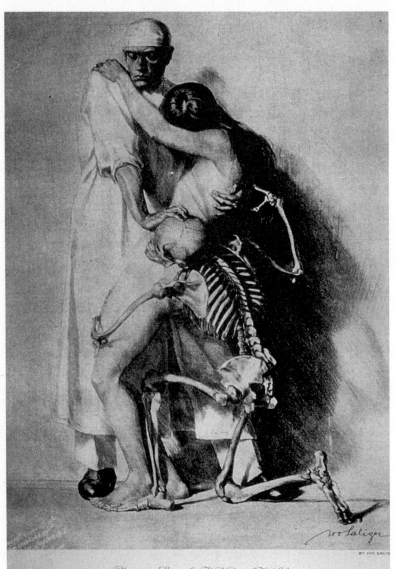

Physician Struggling With Death For Life

EPILOGUE:
FINALLY, JUDGMENT

Pink

"Call the vascular surgery team. Tell them that we are almost ready for them."

I had nearly finished the resection of a bone sarcoma from the proximal fibula.

Carol, the young patient under my care, had already received chemotherapy that had shrunk an initially grapefruit-sized tumor down to the size of a golf ball. As the tumor shrank, it took with it all three major vessels that normally branch into the leg below the knee.

All three --- the anterior tibial, posterior tibial, and peroneal arteries --- were encased in the mass of tumor and scar tissue that was now the proximal fibula. The surgery up to that point convinced me that there was no safe way to free even one of the vessels from the tumor mass.

As the vascular surgery team arrived to build a bypass to reconnect at least one of these vessels across the created gap so that the foot could survive, we completed our resection by tying off the main vessel trunk above where it divides into three branches. Tightening the black silk suture around that last vessel nearly nauseated me. Vascular bypasses, when they are rarely necessary after such tumor resections, have a high failure rate. When they fail, amputation can become inevitable.

"I'll leave this tagged for you, then," I nodded welcome to the vascular surgeon, who had just entered the room. "Thanks for coming down. Obviously, I hoped we wouldn't need your services after all, but thanks for being ready."

"You had to take them all?"

"Yes. This is the popliteal trunk right here. We have the distal posterior tib down here."

"That foot looks awfully pink to be connected to a limb with a tied-off popliteal artery. Are you sure you tied the main trunk?"

I was. The head vascular surgeon didn't scrub into the case, but I showed him all the dissection.

"Maybe she has an anatomic variant with a high popliteal-tibial take-off," he suggested.

"Even with a high take-off, you can see the trunk there. My dissection goes all the way up," I explained.

"I see what you mean, but the foot is pink," he said. "I'm not going to bypass to an already pink foot. Let's get a sterile Doppler up for you to check her pulse."

The nurse brought the wiring and probe for the Doppler, which is an ultrasound probe that will generate an audible signal from a flowing vessel's pulse. She opened it onto the field.

I protested once more: "I have no idea why the foot remains pink. I only know that there's no named vessel connecting from the knee to the foot and ankle."

To use a Doppler, we place a jelly-like substance on the skin near the vessel to be checked. The gel transmits the vibrations from blood flow in the vessel to the probe.

Although the probe picked up no clear pulsatile flow, there was slow, steady blood flow through the vessel.

"Does the foot still feel warm?" the vascular surgeon asked.

"Yes," I said. "It's definitely warm."

"Listen, this may sound crazy, but I think you should close up for now. I want to check her foot again with her in a normal position and with her wound dressings on," the vascular surgeon decided.

We rinsed her wound, finished a minor reconstruction of the

ligaments that stabilize Carol's knee on that side, and sutured her skin closed. After dressings were applied to the wound, the vascular surgeon and I examined Carol's foot again. It remained warm and pink. He tried the Doppler probe again. This time, a very faint pulse was detected in two places. We put another instrument that checks the oxygenation level in the blood onto Carol's big toe. The percentage output read in the low nineties.

"Unbelievable," he said, shaking his head. "Do you have any idea how unlikely that is?"

Not all uncertainty stacks against patients and physicians. Even something as relatively "certain" as anatomy can have variation. All we can guess about Carol's leg is that her named vessels must have been slowly compromised as the tumor grew and shrank back. If their flow was constricted slowly enough, her leg might have used the time as an opportunity to enhance flow through smaller, unnamed collateral vessels in the skin and muscles. This is a fine theory, but I have no real explanation.

As time has proceeded, Carol has continued to improve her blood flow to that foot. She now has even stronger pulses, detectable with fingers rather than a Doppler. She has never needed a bypass.

Other authors have written volumes about inspiring stories of individuals beating the odds, experiencing miracles. I have seen many. Uncertainty fuels these success stories as much as it does the failures of medicine. In my own field of sarcoma surgery, uncertainty remains the only source of hope for some patients.

In this book, you and I have reviewed some of the uncertainties that envelop every patient interacting with even the most modern, technologically advanced medicine. At our best, physicians turn to data from populations to address this uncertainty most safely and predictably. Biology, at work through so much of medical diagnosis, treatment, and prognosis, varies in a predictably broad range, challenging the application of population-based data to an individual.

All biological scientists face these natural population distributions. Physicians especially jumble them because we try not only to learn Nature's laws, but also to manipulate them. We not only *observe* with some statistical percentage of confidence, we *act* and force it to round down to zero percent or round up to one hundred percent.

Nailing it Down

Filling my responsibilities as an educator of physicians-in-training at a medical school, I most frequently work with residents in the third year of their five-year orthopaedic surgical training. Because these residents spend their first year of training mostly away from orthopaedics on other loosely related rotations, they have been in orthopaedics itself for less than two years when they join our sarcoma team. Because of the technical character of orthopaedic knowledge and the fact that medical school studies barely touch on it, they have typically spent their second year overwhelmed as they drank from the fire-hydrant of clinical orthopaedic information. Most third-year residents wake from this second-year reverie and realize that their training years are nearly half-spent, without their having learned much of anything about performing surgical procedures. Many almost panic about the accrual of surgical hand skills at this point.

Their favorite surgery while on our team is the preventative nailing of an impending femur fracture. When a patient with breast, prostate, or some other cancer has developed metastatic disease in the femur, it can elevate the risk of structural failure in the form of fracture. When risk of fracture is high, we will slide a titanium rod down the central canal of the bone to stabilize it and hopefully prevent a break. We use the same implants and general insertion technique as any orthopaedic surgeon would use in fixing a broken femur. The only difference is that this femur isn't broken, only *about* to break.

That fact adds a few minor challenges due to the notion that unbroken bones will not "give" during the insertion of a rigid implant. Otherwise, the unbroken-ness makes it much easier. Residents can see in clear order and run through the mechanical steps of nail insertion. The procedures are prosaic, rather boring really. No one less than obsessed with rote steps and hand skills could find the nailing of an unbroken femur the least bit interesting.

Whenever a third-year resident's eyes light up at the prospect of an upcoming preventative nailing, I cannot help but roll my eyes in response. I remember the feeling from my own time in that position, not all that long ago, but I also know from my experience since how inappropriate my focus on hand skills and steps was. I advise them to stop focusing on maneuvers, hand skills, and surgical steps. This knowledge will naturally develop with even a brief experience in orthopaedics.

I advise them instead to focus on learning surgical judgment. Learn how and when to offer which surgery to which patient. Learn how and when to judge that a given surgical step has been completed with adequate success.

A surgeon with adequate hand skills and excellent judgment will be a great surgeon. A surgeon with gifted, superlative hand skills and poor judgment will be a poor surgeon.

I have known a couple of surgeons possessing truly gifted hands. By couple, I literally mean two. One specialized in hand and forearm surgeries, the other in arthroscopy. Their surgeries were almost beautiful to watch. No struggle. No wasted motion. Tissue planes gracefully leapt out of the hand surgeon's path. Even the more difficult moves with an arthroscope appeared easy when this arthroscopist handled the instruments.

Even for these two surgeons, though, did their superlative skill result from physical talent alone? The surgeries that I performed under their guidance as a trainee were also smoother than they should have been. With their hands off the instruments, their judgment made my hands better. Was it really all hand talent? No.

In the larger part of medicine, in which hand skills don't matter whatsoever, everything comes down to judgment. Good judgment requires knowing all that can be known, knowing where to find the information that isn't stored in memory, and knowing when uncertainty arrives.

Information and access to it expand so rapidly these days that physicians maintain no monopoly on medical knowledge. Good physicians do learn how to sort and judge the wash of information available. They learn how to judge themselves and when reinforcements are needed from another's expertise. That judgment, the judgment when to call in help from another physician, may be the first responsibility of every physician. Beyond it, though, judgment drives the ordering of tests, their interpretation, assembly of treatment options, and education of patients to choose between options, as well as to know what can and cannot be anticipated to follow each.

The critical role of judgment filling in gaps prompts many citizens --- physicians or patients --- to argue about different health care systems. When grays are divided into blacks and whites, who makes those decisions? Population-based evidence enacted into rigid laws? Bureaucratic panels? Physicians? Uneducated patients subjected to advertising or over-educated insurance actuaries pinching pennies?

The space for judgment is large but can be drastically altered by systems. This is why they matter. I don't know which style of system is best. I have strong opinions but can see value in the arguments for and against many kinds of systems. I have happily worked in a few. The key for a patient in any system is to find a physician with the heart of a teacher to lead them through it. These are not so difficult to find.

Every patient seeks a skilled and confident physician. As you pick your physician --- or choose the kind of physician you will be for your patients --- be sure to look for skill at communicating, both listening and teaching. Look for the kind of confidence that includes a willingness to look things up, consult other experts and say, "I don't know." If you want, find or be a physician willing to teach which aspects of care are more and less certain. Flee from any physician --- or the temptation to be a physician --- too arrogant to tolerate questions.

Every physician and patient will make judgments of each other and make judgments together of the decisions facing them. I happily judge, uncertain of how I will be judged in return, that facing uncertainty bravely with my patients is much easier than trying to ignore it. When uncertainty remains shrouded in cobwebs and unspoken secrets, the physician suffers alone in awareness of it, the patient suffers alone experiencing it.

Now What?

Lest you conclude that I have judged medicine too harshly, let me mention a few points at the book's closing.

First, writing about uncertainty in medicine from the vantage point of a musculoskeletal oncologic surgeon may not be entirely fair. While every practitioner and patient in medicine will necessarily experience uncertainty, my patients and I bathe in it daily.

You and I have discussed that information from randomized clinical trials guides surgical practice less than it guides some other disciplines in medicine, but I should acknowledge that my field of surgery for sarcoma-type cancers has almost *no* randomized controlled trials offering useful information. Evidence of any kind other than expert opinion rarely informs my specialty field. While I hope that you now better understand that even the best evidence is flawed in its application to individuals, the lack of evidence *is* worse.

Second, I admit that facing the rampant uncertainties in medicine can easily overwhelm. This failing faith in medicine will encourage some to avoid it entirely. I don't recommend this course to you. Many disappointed by scientifically based medicine have turned to alternative medicine instead. They have not escaped uncertainty in doing so. They have likely encountered even more.

I want you to understand medical uncertainty so that you understand *why* scientific medicine may have disappointed you in your own past as a patient. I want you to understand that your physician may have had no ugly ulterior motive, plotting against your well-being. He may have made no mistake whatsoever. Things may have just not turned out as you both hoped they would.

Third, medicine nets a positive benefit for the patients who use it. It has at least since the discovery of antibiotics. (These provided solutions for many of the problems previously caused by visiting doctors and hospitals.) Subsequent to that critical shift in the balance, the last three-quarters of a century have seen many incremental and even a few quantum-leap advances in medical know-how. Currently, medicine helps many more people than it hurts. I doubt very much that I could practice medicine if I didn't believe that with my heart *and* mind.

I don't write this book to dissuade anyone from seeking professional healthcare services. In receipt of such, most will encounter what I judge to be the most well intentioned group among all professionals. There are a few bad apple charlatans in medicine, but fewer, I think, than in any other profession. Instead, I write this book because I think that we can achieve greater honesty between patients and physicians. We can have a different kind of conversation than we have previously had.

Fourth, the silence by which many physicians address uncertainty remains as a residue from a prior era. Physicians once paternalistically took care of their uninformed patients. The very concepts of patient choice and self-determination were not well developed yet in that era. Instead, physicians emphasized beneficence, or meaning well.

Many patients still wish this system to persist. I anticipate that these patients will always be able to find providers of health care willing to make decisions for them.

A few patients are truly incapable of contributing to the decisions involved in their health care, but very few. I have met many others who simply didn't want to get involved. They wanted me to make decisions for them. I can appreciate this. They *pay* me to make decisions for them.

I don't want to know the details of how my accountant prepares my income tax filing, as long as I know that he is honest about. I don't care to know how my mechanic keeps my car running. As a physician, I am in a service industry. Customer service sometimes means making the important decisions with a smile on my face.

All that said, few of those who hope not to participate in their health care decisions have read this far in this book. I think that *you* want to have a conversation with your physician. I hope this book has empowered you to initiate such a conversation with questions. You are entitled to ask questions of your physician, whether you seek his assistance for a hangnail, the sniffles or a life-threatening cancer.

Don't ask every question at once. Pick *one* you like for a start. Patiently accept that medical uncertainty means that some questions will not find answers. Please also understand that while acknowledging and discussing uncertainty doesn't invite it where it wasn't present before, discussing it also cannot free us from it.

You may have noticed that I offered no conclusions to many of the patient stories we discussed in this book. I have many reasons for not concluding these stories from my patients.

First, I have done everything possible to protect the anonymity of these real people, including changing names and some demographics as well as leaving out story ends.

I have also left story ends out because this book is about improving the process of medicine, not about the outcomes of specific medical decisions. You have read stories from patients with many different conditions and at many different moments in that process. Stories help us understand the weaknesses of the process. Stories encourage me to be honest about those weaknesses. Stories cannot replace science when it comes to understanding the outcomes of specific medical decisions. Science is flawed, but it offers the best information we have to guide decisions.

Finally, I have left out the ends of many patient stories because their uncertain stories have not yet ended. You and I have discussed the uncertainty in their situations. I have discussed the uncertainty with them. The uncertainty didn't disappear.

Honesty can grant me a clear conscience and a good night's sleep as a physician, but in my mornings, uncertainty in medicine remains.

After I see Jeff or Alana or Kate or Brandy on the clinic schedule to be seen for a follow-up appointment, I remain anxiously agitated until I have checked their new scans and confirmed that they have made it another three months without cancer relapsing. I never check my clinic schedule before its day arrives because I *would* lose sleep waiting for these test results. I know that some of these precious patients don't sleep those nights before their visits.

I have no power to change the ongoing uncertainty in my patients' situations. I will be the one to tell them about it. I will be the one to teach them what we can do about it. I will do my best to help them understand what may lie ahead and will witness with them their future unfolding.

Beginning at the End

I began this book telling my story of being sacked by a patient because of what I told him. I want to end with another story of a man who was enabled to trust me while deeply embroiled in uncertainty. In contrast to Carl at the book's opening, this man trusted me because I was fully honest in what I told him.

Robert was referred to me early in my practice with a large mass arising from the bone of his pelvis. Despite its larger-than-softball size, he had noticed it only because of worsening sciatica. He had long had an arthritic spine and the resultant symptoms of waxing and waning irritation in the nerve roots that coalesce into his sciatic nerve. These lancing and burning pains to his leg and foot had come and gone over the years but seemed to have persisted recently. Especially when sitting, his foot would quickly begin to tingle uncomfortably, then go completely numb over a few minutes.

His primary care physician had ordered a spine MRI. This set of images showed the long-standing arthritis of the small joints of his spine, but also a destructive tumor in the pelvic bone to one side. The spine imaging only visualized part of the pelvis mass. His physician referred him for further evaluation under my care. We got additional imaging and arranged for a biopsy of the mass, ultimately rendering a diagnosis of leiomyosarcoma of bone, a rather ominous cancer. The mass extended into the soft-tissues inside and outside of the pelvis into the buttocks, as well as across the large joint between the pelvis bone proper and the lowest bone of the spine, the sacrum.

The mass appeared to be resectable with tumor-free margins. The only problem: Robert was 82 years old and had suffered a heart attack eight years prior, addressed at the time with coronary artery bypass surgery. That surgery had successfully returned Robert, a real estate attorney, not only to his law practice but also to golf, hiking, skiing and enjoying time with his grandchildren.

While functioning adequately, though, Robert's heart could no longer boast of its prior strength. I noticed in my clinic that his pulse felt irregular, following a rhythm known as atrial fibrillation. He returned to his cardiologist for a check-up; I presented his difficult case to our multidisciplinary sarcoma treatment-planning conference.

The medical oncologist in our conference doubted that Robert's heart could tolerate any meaningfully powerful chemotherapy. He preferred not to use lighter-duty regimens unless pushed to do so by the appearance of metastatic nodules to the lung in the future months. Our radiation oncologist considered radiation similarly ineffective as an isolated treatment for a bone sarcoma. The other surgeons agreed that, while high risk, surgery offered the only chance of curing him of the cancer.

Robert and I met again a few days later to exchange the external opinions each had obtained, mine from the conference, his from the cardiologist. His wife and son accompanied him for support and to ask their own questions. Accustomed to high-stakes real estate negotiations and judgments, Robert asked measured but insightful questions. With a brief twinkling wink of his eye, he hesitated, then noted, "I'd like to live, but I'm prepared for the alternative." His hesitation came not from emotion or even fear. He had stopped to glance at his wife, who he knew was most concerned with "the alternative."

Judging that he understood both his situation and quantitative decision-making better than most, I gave him my best guesses at percentages, acknowledging that they were guesses only. We weighed every potential scenario, from doing nothing to doing a 10-hour surgery to remove his tumor. He had brought the news from his cardiologist that while the atrial fibrillation wasn't previously detected, it had resulted from his heart muscle being damaged and tired from injuries sustained nearly a decade earlier during his heart attack. His heart rate was well maintained and ought to be kept so during any surgery, but no other heart intervention was likely to improve his recognized moderate surgical risk. In response to this, I quoted him the highest peri-operative risk of death that I have ever quoted to anyone who had anything other than an immediately life-threatening compilation of injuries.

"The chances are in my favor, albeit slightly," he concluded.

"Yes," I agreed.

"Then let's do it."

We reviewed all the risks one more time. I gave him my mobile phone number to call if any questions or misgivings arose between then and the surgery planned for the next week. All three left smiling, Robert's wife mostly following his lead.

Robert's son called my mobile phone the night before the scheduled surgery to seek my advice. Robert had developed a cough and fever over the preceding couple of days. We canceled the surgery and got Robert in to see his internist, who diagnosed pneumonia. This was treated; Robert rescheduled his surgery for two weeks later. I asked him to come see me in my office two days before to be sure his breathing had truly cleared. It had. We reviewed again the significant risks of his upcoming surgery.

"You're not trying to talk me out of it, are you?" he asked.

"I just want your eyes wide open in your choice."

"They are. I'm ready." On this visit, even his wife looked more comfortable with his decision and the situation overall.

After they left the clinic, I put in a call to the anaesthesiology faculty physician assigned to the case. He was particularly experienced with tough heart cases. He routinely used a newer technology of intra-operative ultrasound to watch the heart throughout surgery as well as balance fluid levels and pressures attentively. After leaving detailed messages on his pager and cell phone, I finished my day, deciding that he would call me if he had any questions.

I ran into this anaesthesiologist the next morning, also on his way to the pre-operative holding area, where Robert would be waiting. He thanked me for the phone messages, saying that he hadn't returned them as he had listened to them later in the evening and was already well acquainted with Robert's case, its risks, etc. He had actually prepared to deliver Robert's anaesthesia for his originally scheduled date, two weeks prior. "It sounds like he understands what he is up against," he said matter-of-factly. "I actually expect that if *we* are careful and *you* are careful, he will get through this relatively smoothly."

I agreed. After all, this was a man with a sick heart that didn't prevent him from golf, downhill skiing and hiking. He had to have greater life reserves than his medical history would suggest.

When the faculty anaesthesiologist opened Robert's room door, allowing me to precede him into the room, I was a little dismayed by what I saw. I don't know who looked more pale with terror, Robert's wife or the junior anaesthesia resident reviewing the medical history with Robert and his family. This resident looked at his attending physician and then at me, as if to ask, "Is this really wise?"

I later learned that this resident had gone home the afternoon before, after being on-call the night before that, thus missing the opportunity to prepare for Robert's case ahead of time. He had grabbed Robert's chart from the door on his way into the room. The resident hadn't imagined that he would be administering anaesthesia to an 82-year-old with a history of severe heart problems during a massive pelvis surgery until he was already staring the large family in the face.

Robert's wife's eyes, wide in fear and frustration, found mine. They seemed to beg for relief.

"What has happened?" I asked, really to anyone in the room.

The resident responded --- or rather blurted out --- unable to hide his own panic, "I think we should cancel. We can get a cardiology consult to risk stratify, or even cardiovert him."

Keenly aware that Robert's family's eyes and ears were following every word, I answered the resident. "Robert has been re-evaluated by his long-standing cardiologist, who, in the opinion of our university cardiology team, was more than qualified to assess him. Neither heart team thought that cardioversion was likely to improve the chronically diseased state of his heart muscle. They consider him optimized already. Is it just his high surgical and anaesthetic risks that bother you?"

"Well, . . . yes," the resident answered.

"He understands his risks," I noted.

Here Robert actually piped in, probably hoping to calm his family. "I also understand my chances if I do nothing --- and I don't particularly like them."

The faculty anaesthesiologist then asked the resident, clearly seeing a teaching moment, "What do you think his peri-operative mortality risk is, given what you have read in his chart?"

"I don't know, maybe as high as 5 percent."

"Well, I signed up for higher than that --- so let's get on with this," Robert said, with his typical wink. His children seemed to relax from his confidence. Even his wife took a seat next to his stretcher, mollified at least.

Whether or not he should have, Robert trusted me. He had prepared himself to face the uncertainties he knew surrounded this day. A large part of his strength derived from his feeling, completely irrationally founded, that I would make sure that our team did our very best for him. I believe that part of his trust came from my acknowledgement up-front of all the vagaries involved in his situation. He trusted we would do our best because he and I had already shared the worst of what we knew, that some things remained uncertain.

REFERENCES

Notes from Chapter 1

1. Exodus chapters 19 through 31 in the Old Testament of the *Bible* comprise multiple visits to the top of Mount Sinai in Horeb, where Moses conversed with God in the form of a burning bush.

2. Although the principle likely pre-dated the man to whom we ascribe it, the history of Occam's razor and its namesake are discussed at length in the Encyclopædia Britannica.

Encyclopædia Britannica Online. 2010. Retrieved 12 June 2010. http://www.britannica.com/EBchecked/topic/424706/Ockhams-razor.

3. Two studies by the same group of investigators reviewed the prevalence of abnormal findings in MRIs of the spine in the neck and the lower back of adults without any related complaints.

Boden SD, McCowin PR, Davis DO, Dina TS, Mark AS, Wiesel S. Abnormal magnetic-resonance scans of the cervical spine in asymptomatic subjects. A prospective investigation. *Journal of Bone and Joint Surgery (American)* 1990;72(8):1178-84. This study identified disc abnormalities in 25 percent of the necks of individuals under forty who were scanned and in 60 percent of individuals over forty. Major abnormalities were found in 19 percent.

Boden SD, Davis DO, Dina TS, Patronas NJ, Wiesel SW. Abnormal magnetic-resonance scans of the lumbar spine in asymptomatic subjects. A prospective investigation. *Journal of Bone and Joint Surgery (American)* 1990;72(3):403-8. There was degeneration or bulging of a disc at one lumbar level in 35 per cent of the subjects between twenty and thirty-nine years old and in all but one of the sixty to eighty-year-old subjects.

4. The Health Insurance Plan (HIP) of New York trial was the first major study of mammography. It began in 1963 and offered annual mammography to women between 40 and 64 years old. It showed a reduction in death from breast cancer by 23-24 percent for all ages screened, but only detected breast cancer by mammography in 6 study patients under 50. Some analyses have found this statistically significant. Others have not. Here is one analysis that found a benefit.

Chu KC, Smart CR, Tarone RE. Analysis of breast cancer mortality by age for the Health Insurance Plan Clinical Trial. *Journal of National Cancer Institute* 1988;80:1125–31.

The Malmö trial invited 21 thousand women over age 45 to screening and followed another 21 thousand in a control group. As a whole, it showed no difference between groups. Five screenings over a decade were performed. The under-55 age group saw a 29 percent increase in death from breast cancer. The over-55 age group saw a 20 percent decrease in death from breast cancer.

Andersson I, Aspegren K, Janzon L, Landberg T, Lindholm K, Linell F, Ljungberg O, Ranstam J, Sigfússon B. Mammographic screening and mortality from breast cancer: the Malmö mammographic screening trial. *British Medical Journal* 1988;297(6654):943-8.

The Two County trial enrolled 133 thousand women from two adjacent counties in Sweden. Multiple reports have come from these parallel cohort studies, with later results at long-term follow-up maintaining the benefit seen early on at a reduction of about 31 percent in deaths from breast cancer.

Tabár L, Fagerberg CJ, Gad A, et al. Reduction in mortality from breast cancer after mass screening with mammography: randomised trial from the Breast Cancer Screening Working Group of the Swedish National Board of Health and Welfare. Lancet 1985;1(8433):829–832.

Tabar L, Fagerberg G, Duffy SW, Day NE. The Swedish Two County Trial of Mammographic Screening for Breast Cancer: Recent Results and Calculation of Benefit. *Journal of Epidemiology and Community Health (1979-)* 1989;43(2):107-114

Tabár L, Vitak B, Chen TH, Yen AM, Cohen A, Tot T, Chiu SY, Chen SL, Fann JC, Rosell J, Fohlin H, Smith RA, Duffy SW. Swedish two-county trial: impact of mammographic screening on breast cancer mortality during 3 decades. *Radiology* 2011;260(3):658-63.

The Edinburgh trial enrolled 44 thousand women and found a not statistically significant reduction of breast cancer mortality of 17 percent overall, but a significant reduction of 20 percent in patients over 50.

Alexander FE, Anderson TJ, Brown HK, Forrest AP, Hepburn W, Kirkpatrick AE, McDonald C, Muir BB, Prescott RJ, Shepherd SM, et al.

The Edinburgh randomised trial of breast cancer screening: results after 10 years of follow-up. *British Journal of Cancer* 1994;70(3):542-8.

The Stockholm trial also found a non-significant reduction of 26 percent in breast cancer mortality overall, but 38 percent significant reduction for women over 50. Women 40 to 49 years old had a non-significant increase in breast cancer mortality of 8 percent.

Frisell J, Lidbrink E, Hellström L, Rutqvist LE. Followup after 11 years --- update of mortality results in the Stockholm mammographic screening trial. *Breast Cancer Research and Treatment* 1997;45(3):263-70.

The Gothenburg trial, a later trial, showed decreased mortality in a young population.

Bjurstam N, Björneld L, Duffy SW, Smith TC, Cahlin E, Eriksson O, Hafström LO, Lingaas H, Mattsson J, Persson S, Rudenstam CM, Säve-Söderbergh J. The Gothenburg breast screening trial: first results on mortality, incidence, and mode of detection for women ages 39-49 years at randomization. *Cancer* 1997;80(11):2091-9.

The Canadian trial, which is considered the most rigorously designed trial, including a control group of patients that undergoes regular clinical examinations, just not mammography, found no added benefit of mammography itself. It was reported in two papers, for two different age groups.

Miller AB, Baines CJ, To T, Wall C. Canadian National Breast Screening Study. I. Breast cancer detection and death rates among women aged 40–49 years. *Canadian Medical Association Journal* 1992; 147:1459-1476.

Miller AB, Baines CJ, To T, Wall C. Canadian National Breast Screening Study. II. Breast cancer detection and death rates among women aged 50–59 years. *Canadian Medical Association Journal* 1992; 147:1477-1488.

The medical literature has numerous opinion papers written on this subject. One of the most often cited is the following. These investigators have rigorously evaluated the quality of the trial designs for each of the above studies, ultimately finding only the Malmö and the Canadian trials as having adequate randomization and control groups, as well as optimal detection and follow-up of cases. They actually conclude that mammography of any kind isn't justified, let alone that for the younger age populations.

Gotzsche PC, Olsen O. Is screening for breast cancer with mammography justifiable? *Lancet* 2000; 355:129-134.

Notes from Chapter 2

1. A number of studies have investigated the sensitivity (ability to detect as positive truly positive cases) and specificity (ability to detect as negative truly negative cases) of the rapid strep test.

Jonckheer T, Goossens H, De Donder M, Levy J, Butzler JP. Evaluation of the direct detection of group A beta-hemolytic streptococcal antigen in a pediatric population: comparison with the traditional culture technique. *European Journal of Epidemiology.* 1986;2(3):205-7. This study found the rapid strep test 81 percent sensitive and 97 percent specific, compared to throat culture as a gold standard.

2. The following article offers a review of the diagnostic criteria for Marfan syndrome that began with completely clinical findings:

Pyeritz, R. E., McKusick, V. A. The Marfan syndrome. *New England Journal of Medicine* 1979;300:772-777.

Medical genetics specialists refer to the criteria for diagnosis of Marfan syndrome in this paper as the "Berlin nosology," because they were discussed and agreed upon at an international conference focused on diagnostic criteria for inherited diseases, which took place in Berlin.

Beighton, P., de Paepe, A., Danks, D., Finidori, G., Gedde-Dahl, T., Goodman, R., Hall, J. G., Hollister, D. W., Horton, W., McKusick, V. A., Opitz, J. M., Pope, F. M., Pyeritz, R. E., Rimoin, D. L., Sillence, D., Spranger, J. W., Thompson, E., Tsipouras, P., Viljoen, D., Winship, I., Young, I. International nosology of heritable disorders of connective tissue. *American Journal of Medical Genetics* 1988;29:581-594.

The next round of internationally agreed upon diagnostic criteria for Marfan syndrome followed a meeting in Ghent, Belgium. These criteria are referred to as the "Ghent nosology." Importantly, these criteria added dural ectasia, a specific finding in the spine to the prior criteria.

De Paepe, A., Devereux, R. B., Dietz, H. C., Hennekam, R. C. M., Pyeritz, R. E. Revised diagnostic criteria for the Marfan syndrome. *American Journal of Medical Genetics* 1996;62: 417-426.

This paper documents the impact of the two different sets of diagnostic criteria on a population of patients under treatment for Marfan syndrome. Almost a quarter of the patients wouldn't have been diagnosed using the Berlin criteria, but were from the Ghent criteria, because of the addition of the spine findings.

Rose, P. S., Levy, H. P., Ahn, N. U., Sponseller, P. D., Magyari, T., Davis, J., Francomano, C. A. A comparison of the Berlin and Ghent nosologies and the influence of dural ectasia in the diagnosis of Marfan syndrome. *Genetics in Medicine* 2000;2:278-282.

3. Dr. James Ewing described the tumor that would eventually bear his name in the following article:

Ewing, J. Diffuse endothelioma of bone. *Proceedings of the New York Pathology Society* 1921;21: 17-24.

The following study marked the beginning of the shift toward defining Ewing sarcoma by its staining with CD99 immunohistochemistry:

Kovar, H., Dworzak, M., Strehl, S., Schnell, E., Ambros, I. M., Ambros, P. F., Gadner, H. Overexpression of the pseudoautosomal gene MIC2 in Ewing's sarcoma and peripheral primitive neuroectodermal tumor. *Oncogene* 1990;5:1067-1070.

The following paper was the first to identify the chromosomal translocation in Ewing's tumors from patients:

Aurias, A., Rimbaut, C., Buffe, D., Zucker, J.M., Mazabraud, A. Translocation involving chromosome 22 in Ewing's sarcoma: a cytogenetic study of four fresh tumors. *Cancer Genetics and Cytogenetics* 1984;12:21-25.

Then, it was found that most Ewing's sarcomas had the specific chromosomal translocation.

Turc-Carel, C., Aurias, A., Mugneret, F., Lizard, S., Sidaner, I., Volk, C., Thiery, J. P., Olschwang, S., Philip, I., Berger, M. P., Philip, T., Lenoir, G. M., Mazabraud, A. Chromosomes in Ewing's sarcoma. I. An evaluation of 85 cases and remarkable consistency of t(11;22)(q24;q12). *Cancer Genetics and Cytogenetics* 1988;32:229-238.

This larger series of patients confirmed the translocation in 95% of Ewing's sarcoma cases.

Lin, P. P., Brody, R. I., Hamelin, A. C., Bradner, J. E., Healey, J. H., Ladanyi, M. Differential transactivation by alternative EWS-FLI1 fusion proteins correlates with clinical heterogeneity in Ewing's sarcoma. *Cancer Research* 1999;59:1428-1432.

This review article discusses the shift in diagnostic strategies from the appearance of tumors under a microscope to the use of specific molecular tests.

Miettinen M. From morphological to molecular diagnosis of soft tissue tumors. *Advances in Experimental Medicine and Biology* 2006;587:99-113.

This report documents some Ewing sarcomas that don't fit the original diagnostic criteria, but would be treated as Ewing sarcoma today due to molecular test results.

Machado I, Noguera R, Mateos EA, Calabuig-Fariñas S, López FI, Martínez A, Navarro S, Llombart-Bosch A. The many faces of atypical Ewing's sarcoma. A true entity mimicking sarcomas, carcinomas and lymphomas. *Virchows Archiv* 2011;458(3):281-90.

4. The original publication of the SLICED study follows:

Skeletal Lesions Interobserver Correlation among Expert Diagnosticians (SLICED) Study Group. Reliability of histopathologic and radiologic grading of cartilaginous neoplasms in long bones. *Journal of Bone and Joint Surgery (American)* 2007;89(10):2113-23.

A second study, on the same topic but with different patient samples and a different group of diagnosticians, these from Europe, was published a couple of years later, reporting similar findings:

Eefting D, Schrage YM, Geirnaerdt MJ, Le Cessie S, Taminiau AH, Bovée JV, Hogendoorn PC; EuroBoNeT consortium. Assessment of interobserver variability and histologic parameters to improve reliability in classification and grading of central cartilaginous tumors. *American Journal of Surgical Pathology* 2009;33(1):50-7.

5. Although John Cameron's emphasis of physician responsibility is admirable, many have investigated the value of CT scans in the setting of possible acute appendicitis since then. Although still controversial, the consensus seems to fall toward favoring CT scans as a means of lowering (definitely not eliminating) the rate of surgical removal of what turn out to be normal appendices. The following article reviews the data from a number of studies in a systematic fashion:

Krajewski S, Brown J, Phang PT, Raval M, Brown CJ. Impact of computed tomography of the abdomen on clinical outcomes in patients with acute right lower quadrant pain: a meta-analysis. *Canadian Journal of Surgery* 2011;54(1):43-53.

6. The following three articles report on three studies that measured the impact of multi-disciplinary tumor boards on patient care decisions and outcomes.

Greer HO, Frederick PJ, Falls NM, Tapley EB, Samples KL, Kimball KJ, Kendrick JE, Conner MG, Novak L, Straughn JM Jr. Impact of a weekly multidisciplinary tumor board conference on the management of women with gynecologic malignancies. *International Journal of Gynecological Cancer* 2010;20(8):1321-5.

Wheless SA, McKinney KA, Zanation AM. A prospective study of the clinical impact of a multidisciplinary head and neck tumor board. *Otolaryngology, Head and Neck Surgery* 2010;143(5):650-4.

Newman EA, Guest AB, Helvie MA, Roubidoux MA, Chang AE, Kleer CG, Diehl KM, Cimmino VM, Pierce L, Hayes D, Newman LA, Sabel MS. Changes in surgical management resulting from case review at a breast cancer multidisciplinary tumor board. *Cancer* 2006;107(10):2346-51.

7. Two very large studies have been reported, each arguing against the value of PSA screening for men.

Andriole GL, Crawford ED, Grubb RL 3rd, Buys SS, Chia D, Church TR, Fouad MN, Gelmann EP, Kvale PA, Reding DJ, Weissfeld JL, Yokochi LA, O'Brien B, Clapp JD, Rathmell JM, Riley TL, Hayes RB, Kramer BS, Izmirlian G, Miller AB, Pinsky PF, Prorok PC, Gohagan JK, Berg CD; PLCO Project Team. Mortality results from a randomized prostate-cancer screening trial. *New England Journal of Medicine* 2009 Mar 26;360(13):1310-9. This study reported no difference in prostate cancer-related deaths in the 38,000 men screened compared to an equally large control group.

Schröder FH, Hugosson J, Roobol MJ, Tammela TL, Ciatto S, Nelen V, Kwiatkowski M, Lujan M, Lilja H, Zappa M, Denis LJ, Recker F, Berenguer A, Määttänen L, Bangma CH, Aus G, Villers A, Rebillard X, van der Kwast T, Blijenberg BG, Moss SM, de Koning HJ, Auvinen A; ERSPC Investigators. Screening and prostate-cancer mortality in a randomized European study. *New England Journal of Medicine* 2009 Mar 26;360(13):1320-8. This study, published in the exact same issue of the New England Journal of Medicine, reported a reduction in prostate cancer specific mortality of 20 percent in the screened population of 182,000 men, but a great increase in overdiagnosis and its expected problems, given morbid treatments available. Only one death was prevented for every 48 additional men treated for prostate cancer.

This third study estimates actual rates of overdiagnosis and the specific numerical value of lead-time bias from PSA screening in men.

Telesca D, Etzioni R, Gulati R. Estimating lead time and overdiagnosis associated with PSA screening from prostate cancer incidence trends. *Biometrics* 2008;64(1):10-9. Their results indicate an average lead time of 5 to 7 years and overdiagnosis frequencies of approximately 23 to 33 percent.

Notes from Chapter 3

1. In their working paper number 12436 from the National Bureau of Economic Research in 2006, David Autor and Mark Duggan reported that the percentage of the United States population currently supported by Social Security Disability Insurance rose from 2.2 percent in 1985 to 4.1 percent in 2005. The Social Security Administration paid out 85 billion dollars in 2005 to recipients of disability benefits. This comprised 17 percent of its overall spending. This cost ignores the cost of life-long Medicare supported healthcare for those on disability, beginning two years after the designated date of disability. Summary of this report was retrieved from http://www.nber.org/aginghealth/fall06/w12436.html on 3 October 2011.

Worker's compensation is administered through state and private programs rather than federally/publicly run programs like Social Security Disability. The National Academy of Social Insurance in Washington, DC published a report on 26 August 2008 by Ishita Sengupta, Virginia Reno, and John F. Burton, Jr. that calculated 87.6 billion dollars in total cost of United States employers in 2006, with 26.5 billion of that going toward paying health care costs for injured workers and 28.2 billion going toward wage replacement benefits. That adds up to $1.58 out of every $100 spent on workers total. This report is available at the following address: http://www.nasi.org/usr_doc/NASI_Workers_Comp_Report_2006.pdf

2. What became known as the Waddell signs of incongruity, or a psychological component to back pain, were published in the following report:

Waddell G, McCulloch JA, Kummel E, Venner RM. Nonorganic physical signs in low-back pain. *Spine (Phila Pa 1976)* 1980 Mar-Apr;5(2):117-25.

Dr. Waddell published this later paper reviewing some of the psychology behind these "nonorganic" signs of psychological distress.

Waddell G, Main CJ, Morris EW, Di Paola M, Gray IC. Chronic low-back pain, psychologic distress, and illness behavior. *Spine (Phila Pa 1976)* 1984 Mar;9(2):209-13.

Notes from Chapter 4

1. Lipitor was the single most prescribed drug in the United States in 2005, with sales upwards of 16 billion that year according to data from IMS Health, Annual Report on prescription drug trends (Feb 20, 2006). www.imshealth.com.

2. A search on PubMed on 3 October 2011 yielded more than 4000 articles for the term "placebo effect," ranging from 1953 to the present. The following two are pertinent examples.

Beecher HK (1955). "The powerful placebo". J Am Med Assoc 159 (17): 1602–6.

Hróbjartsson A, Gøtzsche PC. "Is the placebo powerless? An analysis of clinical trials comparing placebo with no treatment". *New England Journal of Medicine* 2001;344(21): 1594–1602.

In addition, more than 4000 books on the subject surface from an Amazon.com search on the same day. Certainly, many of these hits are different editions of the same books, but even 50 books on the topic would be more than enough for us to take notice, one would think.

3. The original publication of what has later been termed the "VA arthroscopy study" was the following:

Moseley JB, O'Malley K, Petersen NJ, Menke TJ, Brody BA, Kuykendall DH, Hollingsworth JC, Ashton CM, Wray NP. A controlled trial of arthroscopic surgery for osteoarthritis of the knee. *New England Journal of Medicine* 2002;347(2):81-8.

4. The following article reports a summary analysis of 36 different trials comparing these different devices for the fixation of what are called extra-capsular hip fractures or intertrochanteric hip fractures.

Parker MJ, Handoll HH. Gamma and other cephalocondylic intramedullary nails versus extramedullary implants for extracapsular hip fractures in adults. *Cochrane Database Systematic Reviews 2008*;(3):CD000093.

5. The 1999 report "To Err is Human" from the United States Institute of

Medicine can be found at the following web address: http://www.nap.edu/openbook.php?isbn=0309068371

6. Sickle-cell anemia was first noted in a patient in 1910 in the following article:

> Herrick JB. Peculiar elongated and sickle-shaped red blood corpuscles in a case of severe anemia. *Archives of Internal Medicine* 1910;6:517–521.

Although the first account described the sickle-shaped red blood cells, the name "sickle cell anemia" came in 1922 from

> Mason VR. Sickle cell anemia. *JAMA* 1922;79(14):1318–1320.

Sickle-cell anemia later became the very first molecular disease in 1949, when Linus Pauling traced the abnormality to a genetic defect in the hemoglobin gene. To put this in perspective, the structure of DNA wasn't even known until 1953, four years later:

> Pauling, Linus; Harvey A. Itano, S. J. Singer, Ibert C. Wells. Sickle Cell Anemia, a Molecular Disease. *Science* 1949;110(2865):543–548.

7. The two initial publications of the Women's Health Initiative that completely changed the thinking regarding hormone replacement therapy are the following:

> Rossouw JE, Anderson GL, Prentice RL, et al. Risks and benefits of estrogen plus progestin in healthy postmenopausal women: principal results From the Women's Health Initiative randomized controlled trial. *JAMA* 2002;288(3):321–33.

> Anderson GL, Limacher M, Assaf AR, et al. Effects of conjugated equine estrogen in postmenopausal women with hysterectomy: the Women's Health Initiative randomized controlled trial. *JAMA* 2004;291(14):1701–12.

8. This review article details the history of the rise of bisphosphonates, initially for use with osteoporosis and then for use in managing cancer metastasis to the bone.

> Fleisch H. Development of bisphosphonates. *Breast Cancer Research* 2002;4(1):30–4.

This article reviews the emerging data about the unusual femur shaft fractures following long-term dosing of bisphosphonates.

> Shane E. Evolving data about subtrochanteric fractures and bisphosphonates. *New England Journal of Medicine* 2010;362(19):1825–7.

9. This is one of the many articles voicing serious questions about the validity of the use of steroids for acute spinal cord injury, promulgated by the National Acute Spinal Cord Injury Studies (NASCISs)

> Nesathurai S. Steroids and spinal cord injury: revisiting the NASCIS 2 and NASCIS 3 trials. *Journal of Trauma* 1998 Dec;45(6):1088-93.

The following three articles are the primary reports of each of the three NASCI studies:

Bracken MB, Shepard MJ, Hellenbrand KG, Collins WF, Leo LS, Freeman DF, Wagner FC, Flamm ES, Eisenberg HM, Goodman JH, et al. Methylprednisolone and neurological function 1 year after spinal cord injury. Results of the National Acute Spinal Cord Injury Study. *Journal of Neurosurgery* 1985;63(5):704-13.

Bracken MB, Shepard MJ, Collins WF, Holford TR, Young W, Baskin DS, Eisenberg HM, Flamm E, Leo-Summers L, Maroon J. A randomized, controlled trial of methylprednisolone or naloxone in the treatment of acute spinal-cord injury. Results of the Second National Acute Spinal Cord Injury Study. *New England Journal of Medicine* 1990;322:1405-11.

Bracken MB, Shepard MJ, Holford TR, Leo-Summers L, Aldrich EF, Fazl M. Administration of methylprednisolone for 24 or 48 hours or tirilazad mesylate for 48 hours in the treatment of acute spinal cord injury. Results of the Third National Acute Spinal Cord Injury Randomized Controlled Trial. National Acute Spinal Cord Injury Study. *JAMA* 1997;277:1597-604.

10. The following four trials with their spiffy names provided the boom and ultimately the bust for wide-spread use of COX2 selective inhibitors and then the company's retraction of rofecoxib (Vioxx):

Silverstein FE, Faich G, Goldstein JL, et al. Gastrointestinal toxicity with celecoxib vs nonsteroidal anti-inflammatory drugs for osteoarthritis and rheumatoid arthritis: the CLASS study: A randomized controlled trial. Celecoxib Long-term Arthritis Safety Study. *JAMA* 2000;284(10):1247–55.

Bombardier C, Laine L, Reicin A, et al. Comparison of upper gastrointestinal toxicity of rofecoxib and naproxen in patients with rheumatoid arthritis. VIGOR Study Group. *New England Journal of Medicine* 2000;343(21):1520–8, 2p following 1528.

Singh G, Fort JG, Goldstein JL, Levy RA, Hanrahan PS, Bello AE, Andrade-Ortega L, Wallemark C, Agrawal NM, Eisen GM, Stenson WF, Triadafilopoulos G; SUCCESS-I Investigators . Celecoxib versus naproxen and diclofenac in osteoarthritis patients: SUCCESS-I Study. *American Journal of Medicine* 2006;119(3):255-66.

Lisse JR, Perlman M, Johansson G, Shoemaker JR, Schechtman J, Skalky CS, Dixon ME, Polis AB, Mollen AJ, Geba GP; ADVANTAGE Study Group. Gastrointestinal tolerability and effectiveness of rofecoxib versus naproxen in the treatment of osteoarthritis: a randomized, controlled trial. *Annals of Internal Medicine* 2003;139(7):539-46.

11. First article reporting measurement of the pump head phenomenon:

Newman M, Kirchner J, Phillips-Bute B, Gaver V, Grocott H, Jones R,

Mark D, Reves J, Blumenthal J. Longitudinal assessment of neurocognitive function after coronary-artery bypass surgery. *New England Journal of Medicine* 2001;344(6):395-402.

Two subsequent articles that argued that non-operative control groups were just as bad, suggesting that pump head may be the natural history of patients with heart disease.

McKhann GM, Grega MA, Borowicz LM Jr, Bailey MM, Barry SJ, Zeger SL, Baumgartner WA, Selnes OA. Is there cognitive decline 1 year after CABG? Comparison with surgical and nonsurgical controls. *Neurology* 2005;65(7):991-9.

Selnes OA, Grega MA, Borowicz LM Jr, Barry S, Zeger S, Baumgartner WA, McKhann GM. Cognitive outcomes three years after coronary artery bypass surgery: a comparison of on-pump coronary artery bypass graft surgery and nonsurgical controls. *Annals of Thoracic Surgery* 2005;79(4):1201-9.

Three articles measuring pump head phenomenon in patients undergoing open heart surgery on or off the bypass pump. The first found that off-pump surgery protected cognition. The second found an improvement only in short-term cognition, which disappeared by a year. The third showed no difference at all.

Zamvar V, Williams D, Hall J, Payne N, Cann C, Young K, Karthikeyan S, Dunne J. Assessment of neurocognitive impairment after off-pump and on-pump techniques for coronary artery bypass graft surgery: prospective randomised controlled trial. *British Medical Journal* 2002;325(7375):1268.

Van Dijk D, Jansen EW, Hijman R, Nierich AP, Diephuis JC, Moons KG, Lahpor JR, Borst C, Keizer AM, Nathoe HM, Grobbee DE, De Jaegere PP, Kalkman CJ; Octopus Study Group.Cognitive outcome after off-pump and on-pump coronary artery bypass graft surgery: a randomized trial. *JAMA* 2002;287(11):1405-12.

Jensen BO, Hughes P, Rasmussen LS, Pedersen PU, Steinbrüchel DA. Cognitive outcomes in elderly high-risk patients after off-pump versus conventional coronary artery bypass grafting: a randomized trial. *Circulation* 2006;113(24):2790-5.

12. Ernest Amory Codman's story is recorded in a number of venues. A brief biography is available on the New England Shoulder and Elbow Surgeons society page, last checked 3 October 2011:

http://www.neses.com/news.article.10.3.2009.php

Codman's own book about the End-Result concept, really a manifesto of sorts, was printed privately, but can be accessed in older library collections.

Codman, Ernest A. (1916). A Study in Hospital Efficiency. Boston: Privately printed.

The most complete biography of the man and his illustrious career is the following:
Mallon, Bill (2000). Ernest Amory Codman: The End Result of a Life in
Medicine. Philadelphia: WB Saunders. ISBN 0-7216-8461-0.

Notes from Chapter 5

1. Some of the history of Richard Johnston is recorded in the following article:
Callaghan JJ. Richard C. Johnston, M.D. evaluator and practitioner of hip
surgery. *Iowa Orthopaedic Journal.* 1996;16:xii-xix.

2. The entire book might have focused on the problem of preventing clot formation in post-operative patients and all the research problems it introduces. The
following are the most recent "evidence-based" guidelines from the American
College of Chest Physicians, mandating what surgeons should do to prevent
clots. The second article is a response of surgeons to the character of the data
as entirely dependent on surrogates.

Jack Hirsh, Gordon Guyatt, Gregory W. Albers, Robert Harrington, and
Holger J. Schünemann. Executive Summary: American College of Chest
Physicians Evidence-Based Clinical Practice Guidelines (8th Edition). *Chest*
2008;133:6 suppl 71S-109S

Weber KL, Zuckerman JD, Watters WC 3rd, Turkelson CM. Deep vein
thrombosis prophylaxis. *Chest* 2009;136(6):1699-700.

3. The large randomized controlled trial that finally confirmed the mortality
benefit of aspirin use following a heart attack follows:

ISIS-2 (Second International Study of Infarct Survival) Collaborative
Group. Randomised trial of intravenous streptokinase, oral aspirin, both,
or neither among 17,187 cases of suspected acute myocardial infarction:
ISIS-2. *Lancet.* 1988 Aug 13;2(8607):349-60.

Earlier trials such as these below had shown no statistically significant difference.
Elwood PC, Sweetnam PM. Aspirin and secondary mortality after myocardial infarction. *Lancet* 1979;2(8156-8157):1313-5.

An intervention study-the aspirin myocardial infarction study. *Lipids*
1977;12(1):59-63.

The Coronary Drug Project Research Group. Aspirin in coronary heart
disease. *Journal of Chronic Disease* 1976;29(10):625-42.

4. Stephen Katz presented at the annual meeting of the American Orthopaedic
Association in June 13-16 2007 in Asheville, North Carolina. The following
article arose from this same symposium, but left out the delightful details of his
question to the audience about whether there is evidence that the orthopaedic
community has used any evidence provided by NIH studies to change their
decision-making:

Marsh JL, McMaster W, Parvizi J, Katz SI, Spindler K. AOA Symposium. Barriers (threats) to clinical research. *Journal of Bone and Joint Surgery (American)* 2008;90(8):1769-76.

5. Decision Analysis has been used in many fields of medicine in the last decade. The article specifically discussed in detail is the following:

Schultz WR, Weinstein JN, Weinstein SL, Smith BG. Prophylactic pinning of the contralateral hip in slipped capital femoral epiphysis: evaluation of long-term outcome for the contralateral hip with use of decision analysis. *Journal of Bone and Joint Surgery (American)* 2002;84(8):1305-14.

The decision analysis that followed the first article by a couple of years, but generated the exactly opposite conclusion is the following:

Kocher MS, Bishop JA, Hresko MT, Millis MB, Kim YJ, Kasser JR. Prophylactic pinning of the contralateral hip after unilateral slipped capital femoral epiphysis. *Journal of Bone and Joint Surgery (American)* 2004;86(12):2658-65.

Announcement of the 2010 DAS Practice Award by the Decision Analysis Society to the Chevron corporation was found at http://www.informs.org/Recognize-Excellence/Community-Prizes-and-Awards/Decision-Analysis-Society/DAS-Practice-Award, last confirmed 3 October 2011.

Notes from Chapter 6

1. A number of articles chronicle the history of chemotherapeutic treatments for osteosarcoma. The following particular citation is an article published by one of the first practitioners using chemotherapy in this setting:

Jaffe N. The potential for an improved prognosis with chemotherapy in osteogenic sarcoma. *Clinical Orthopaedics and Related Research.* 1975;(113):111-8.

2. James N. Weinstein organized the 11-center clinical trial called the Spine Patient Outcomes Research Trial (SPORT). Results from this trial have been published in the *New England Journal of Medicine* and the *Journal of the American Medical Association.* Its initial design is described in the following article:

Birkmeyer NJ, Weinstein JN, Tosteson AN, Tosteson TD, Skinner JS, Lurie JD, Deyo R, Wennberg JE. Design of the Spine Patient outcomes Research Trial (SPORT). *Spine (Phila Pa 1976).* 2002;27(12):1361-72.

Dr. Weinstein has published additional studies on the process of educating patients and has spoken broadly about the topic, based on his experiences in this trial of operative versus non-operative treatment. Additional pertinent references include the following:

Weinstein JN, Clay K, Morgan TS. Informed patient choice: patient-centered valuing of surgical risks and benefits. *Health Aff (Millwood).* 2007 May-Jun;26(3):726-30.

Lurie JD, Spratt KF, Blood EA, Tosteson TD, Tosteson AN, Weinstein

JN. Effects of Viewing an Evidence-Based Video Decision Aid on Patients' Treatment Preferences for Spine Surgery. *Spine (Phila Pa 1976)* 2011;36(18):1501-4.

3. Samuel de Sorbiere's book is quoted in translation in the following book about the history of informed consent:

Katz J. New York, New York: The Free Press, Macmillan, Inc.; 1984. *The Silent World of Doctor and Patient.*

4. Details of the California 1972 court case Canterbury v. Spence are recorded, along with extracts from the judicial briefs, in the following book about the history of informed consent:

Faden RR, Beauchamp TL, King NMP. New York, New York: Oxford University Press; 1986. *A History and Theory of Informed Consent.*

5. This particular passage from *Whitejacket* is in chapter 63. This chapter was available for review at http://www.online-literature.com/view.php/white-jacket/63, last confirmed on 3 October 2011. Paper prints of the book can be found in older library collections.

Notes from Chapter 7

1. The specific study quoted to have reported three of 21 patients surviving to discharge is one of very few articles on the topic of terminal extubation that provides any data beyond opinion, even if it is only observational data.

O'Mahony S, McHugh M, Zallman L, Selwyn P. Ventilator withdrawal: procedures and outcomes. Report of a collaboration between a critical care division and a palliative care service. *Journal of Pain Symptom Management* 2003;26(4):954-61.

The only larger study noted 6 patients surviving to hospital discharge after 166 terminal extubations in 15 ICUs in Canada.

Cook D, Rocker G, Marshall J, Sjokvist P, Dodek P, Griffith L, Freitag A, Varon J, Bradley C, Levy M, Finfer S, Hamielec C, McMullin J, Weaver B, Walter S, Guyatt G; Level of Care Study Investigators and the Canadian Critical Care Trials Group. Withdrawal of mechanical ventilation in anticipation of death in the intensive care unit. *New England Journal of Medicine* 2003 Sep 18;349(12):1123-32.

The Karen Ann Quinlan story can be read in many textbooks and websites dedicated to the "Right to Die" movement, but is recorded in greatest detail by her parents:

Quinlan, J and Quinlan, J. D. (1977). *Karen Ann: The Quinlans Tell Their Story.* New York: Bantam Books. ISBN 0-385-12666-2

2. The following report details the case of a man who awoke fully and returned home after he was declared dead at the end of a session of CPR:

Ben-David B, Stonebraker VC, Hershman R, Frost CL, Williams HK. Survival after failed intraoperative resuscitation: a case of "Lazarus syndrome". *Anesthesia and Analgesia* 2001;92(3):690-2.

The following articles review cases previously reported in the literature of Lazarus syndrome:

Wiese CH, Bartels UE, Orso S, Graf BM. [Lazarus phenomenon. Spontaneous return of circulation after cardiac arrest and cessation of resuscitation attempts]. *Anaesthesist* 2010;59(4):333-41.

Hornby K, Hornby L, Shemie SD. A systematic review of auto-resuscitation after cardiac arrest. *Critical Care Medicine* 2010;38(5):1246–53.

3. The legend of Aesculapius is recorded in many venues. Some direct references to a mortal physician by this name can be found in Homer's *Iliad* itself. One version of the legend can be found in the following reference text:

Hamilton, Edith (1942 --- New edition 1998). Mythology. Back Bay Books. ISBN 0-316-34151-7.

4. The natural history study of scoliosis was reported as the following:

Weinstein SL, Dolan LA, Spratt KF, Peterson KK, Spoonamore MJ, Ponseti IV: Health and function of patients with untreated idiopathic scoliosis: A 50 year natural history study. *JAMA* 2003;289:559-567.

5. Although none approaches 50-year results, the following report the longest-term outcomes of scoliosis fusion surgery. All are from Sweden.

Danielsson AJ, Nachemson AL. Radiological findings and curve progression 22 years after treatment for adolescent idiopathic scoliosis: Comparison of brace and surgical treatment with a matching control group of straight individuals. *Spine* 2001;26:516-525.

Danielsson AJ, Nachemson AL. Childbearing, curve progression, and sexual function in women 22 years after treatment for adolescent idiopathic scoliosis. A case-control study. *Spine* 2001;26:1449-1456.

Danielsson A, Wiklund I, Pehrsson K, Nachemson A. Health-related quality of life in patients with adolescent idiopathic scoliosis: A matched follow up at least 20 years after treatment with brace or surgery. *European Spine Journal* 2001;10:278-288.

Notes from Chapter 8

1. The following is a website dedicated to the biography and writings of John Graunt, curated by a historian focused on the Graunt heritage, last checked 3 October 2011. The website includes images from Graunt's report on the Bills of Mortality.

http://www.edstephan.org/Graunt/graunt.html

2. Weiss Ratings 2004 report noted that the Life Insurance industry averages 8.2 percent profit margins.

3. This study from Dartmouth makes clear the massive effects on death by many causes for a population that smokes. So drastic is the impact that the epidemiologists at Dartmouth had to make two separate tables for causes of death among smokers and non-smokers:

Woloshin S, Schwartz LM, Welch HG. Risk charts: putting cancer in context. *Journal of the National Cancer Institute* 2002;94(11):799-804.

4. Health care expenditures in the United States of America as estimated by the Office of the Actuary, The Centers for Medicare and Medicaid services are available at https://www.cms.gov/NationalHealthExpendData/02_National HealthAccountsHistorical.asp#TopOfPage, last checked on 3 October 2011, these showed only 2009 numbers at the latest, with 2.49 trillion total health care expenditures in the United States for that year

5. Although people throw the consideration around liberally in conversation, the actual expenditures during the last two weeks of life have not been the focus of much detailed study to the best of my knowledge. Medicare estimates that nearly a third of its annual costs go toward expenditures during the last year of life, according to an article on 19 October 2006 by Julie Appleby in the *USA Today* newspaper. Actual expenditures during the last week of life (much smaller numbers than are actually thrown around routinely in political conversation) have been found to change dependent on conversations individuals have had with their families and physicians about end-of-life issues.

Zhang B, Wright AA, Huskamp HA, Nilsson ME, Maciejewski ML, Earle CC, Block SD, Maciejewski PK, Prigerson HG. Health care costs in the last week of life: associations with end-of-life conversations. *Archives of Internal Medicine* 2009;169(5):480-8.

Notes from Chapter 9

1. The Terri Schiavo case has been recorded by many authors and journalists. Most records have some axe to grind. There are more than 370 books on Amazon that come up from a search of her name alone. To skeleton the events for the purpose of our discussion, I used Wikipedia, last checked on 3 October 2011, with the hope that its open format might balance the many opinions about her story. Most of the dates and details are also available in the public records of the state of Florida.

Please find links to these references as well as additional information at:

www.DoctorsCannotTellYou.com/RawData

ACKNOWLEDGEMENTS

I owe a heavy debt of gratitude to my family for giving me the time to write this book. Adding writing time on top of my more-than-full-time scientific and surgical professional pursuits did not *only* steal from my sleeping hours. Ever supportive, my wife has served as listener, reader, and trusted advisor. My youngest child insists on repeating the book's title to everyone he meets, almost to prove that he is "big" enough to speak the words. My oldest writes and crayon-illustrates her "books" at a pace I will never match. The middle two children ask for only occasional breaks from my work to kick a soccer ball or read another book aloud.

Many of the ideas for this book derived from conversations during my residency training in orthopaedics with Joseph A. Buckwalter, mentor and friend, and conversations over the last three years with Samuel Brown, my peer in age, but my far-superior in intellect and wisdom.

Writing text intended to be readable and enjoyable for both physicians and non-physicians proved a task more difficult than I first supposed. You will judge how successful I was at it, but whatever I accomplished in that regard, I accomplished not alone but with the helpful responses of many readers of early

drafts, including but not limited to Sheila Barnett, Russell and
Marilyn McSweeney, Catherine Edwards, Steve Kelly, Bruce
and Jo Ann Jones, Ernie and Nancy Ewin, Carol Lenz, Sebrena
Banecker, Holly Spraker, Carol and Paul Garza, Barbara and
Leslie Moon, Nancy Bender, Marianne Bowling, R. Lor Randall,
Charles Saltzman, Ingrid Nygaard, Janie and Ed Rogers,
Candace Seedall, Richard Call, Kim Wilson, Greg Monson,
Nicholas and Krystal Straessler, Michael Potter, George Calvert,
Martin Ehman, Hailey Fitzgerald, Carrie Hickman, Katie
Thomas, Hal and Pam Cole, Joseph Buckwalter, Rick Focht,
Catalina and Victoria Ritzinger, Mary Hofheins, Jim Thornton,
Rob Koeliker, Sam Green, Paige Peterson, Lori Kun, and Susan
Sheehan.

I offer specific thanks to Matthew Wade Bradley (1970-2012),
who proved a critically helpful reader and inspiring friend.
His story proves the inexroable uncertainty of medicine: after
surviving what should have been a deadly cancer, his young life
was taken by a completely unanticipated accident the very week
this book went to press. He will be remembered fondly by many.

Finally, I gratefully acknowledge my patients. I learn so much
from them. Even Carl, who fired me, taught me more than
he can possibly realize about the fragile interactions between
physicians and patients. I do not begrudge him in the slightest.
I involve myself in patient care because I am constantly
humbled and delighted by the privileged glimpses into life that
medicine affords me. Certainly, I am grateful for the patients
depicted in these stories, but I am no less grateful for the many
whose stories remain untold beyond our private, privileged
conversations.